Martica K Heaner, originally from Texas, has lived in London for several years. She was awarded UK 1992 Fitness Leader of the Year and nominated for an award for Special Achievement in the Fitness Industry in 1994. She was a British Aerobics Champion Silver Medallist in 1989 and is certified by ACE and AFAA. She writes regularly for many leading magazines and newspapers. She is also featured on the bestselling video, 'Thighs, Tums and Bums'.

GW00697100

CURVES

The Body Transformation Strategy

Martica K Heaner

Hodder & Stoughton

First published in Great Britain in 1995 by Hodder and Stoughton Ltd
A division of Hodder Headline Plc

10 9 8 7 6 5 4 3 2 1

ISBN 0 340 63866 4

Printed and bound in Great Britain by
BPC Hazell Books Ltd, Aylesbury, Bucks

Hodder and Stoughton Ltd
A Division of Hodder Headline PLC
338 Euston Road,
London NW1 3BH

Photography:

Cover Photo:	Graham Tucker
Hair and Make-up:	Janice Tee, London
Inside Pictures:	(Stretches) Select Studios, Houston
	(Conditioning Exercises) Graham Tucker, London
Cover Leotard:	Sport Europa
Shoes:	Avia
Weights:	Energy Express

For my Grandmother, Beatrice Loock Heaner,
and my friend, Sally Wadyka

Acknowledgements

I want to thank Darley Anderson and Patricia Taylor for believing in me, Rowena Webb for making that belief a reality, Kathy and David Hannah, Harwood (Billy) Taylor for an inspirational brainstorming session, Shelley Marks and Jenni Baden for encouragement, Dr Nick Walters at the University of Westminster, and Jenna Seiden for proofreading the book, Cannons Sports Clubs, The Metropolitan Group, Peter Lawson and Simon Rutter at Avia UK, and Fitness Professionals for their support.

Contents

PART ONE

THE LEARNING CURVE

There are four sections in this book:

- Part One will explain the Body Transformation Strategy to show you exactly what you need to do to reach your goal.

- Part Two will show you how to choose the right activities for you by taking the four 'Ps' into account: your personality, your psychology, your physical needs and your practical requirements.

- Part Three will give you specific Body Transformation Curves to follow.

- Part Four will show you how to stay motivated to ensure that you stick to your fitness plan.

CHAPTER 1

The Problem

I became an aerobics instructor at the start of the American fitness boom. The fitness craze was still in its developmental stages when I arrived in the UK some years later. Throughout my teaching in both countries I've come across thousands of people on the quest for self-improvement – people of all shapes, sizes, ages and nationalities. As a health journalist for many years I've also received letters from all types of readers. But, as different as these people are, there is something most of them have in common. Their mistakes.

In the hope of transforming their body many of them blindly try each new exercise trend or fad diet. Very few are successful. After a lot of self-denial and frustration, most people are the same body weight and shape they were when they *started* the compulsive regimens two, five or ten years ago. Some are even worse off.

Even those who aren't concerned with their body *shape*, but who exercise for other reasons, don't necessarily reach their goal. Take the case of Jim Fixx, the guru credited with spurring the running craze. He ran serious distances to improve his health. He was on the right track, but didn't follow the exact exercise prescription he should have for his pre-existing heart condition. So when he had a headline-making heart attack and died, his mistake provided invaluable fodder for hordes of self-righteous, non-exercising types. But the lesson to be learned is not 'running is bad for you', but 'run as often and as hard as is *suited to your individual fitness level*'.

Look at the many people who exercise to improve their fitness. Due to a lack of knowledge about *what* to do or *how* to do it, they often do the wrong type of exercise for their needs, or follow poor advice from an unqualified coach or teacher. It's no surprise when they hurt their back or knees – *permanently*.

Even many of those frantic, Type A personalities who hear that exercise relieves stress may try a fitness activity or sport, then be so sore the next day that their stress release is negligible. Or they may join a health club, have one mind-boggling aerobics class, then decide to watch TV to relax instead. They have the right idea but the wrong approach.

That's not to say the health boom has been littered with nothing but failure. There have been many success stories too. But too often these are short-lived. In fact, so many people drop out after beginning a self-improvement health programme of diet and/ or exercise that a whole field of research has evolved dedicated to studying what motivates people and what makes them adhere to a regimen. Even those who experience some gains have often found them to be only temporary. Despite fleeting success they, too, have followed the same blind path towards fitness.

Dropping Out

Different people with different goals make the same mistake over and over again. Sadly, most of these people aren't even aware that their failure and wasted time can be avoided. And usually they never realise that they are doingsomething wrong. As a result, many give up. Nobody likes to fail, so why bother?

The problem is, when you drop out, you're *guaranteed* not to see any results.

Trying Anything and Everything

Others persist, especially women who feel the nagging social pressure to retain beauty and youth. The fact is, the numerous methods available are obviously not very effective because people keep trying new ones. People keep buying *more* diet books, *more* fitness videos, trying out *more* treatments, lotions and potions in the attempt to make their bodies beautiful. This compulsion perpetuates *more* quack cures and fad diets. And *more* failure. After a while they all blend into one big, empty promise.

Failure Leads to Rebellion

At the very least, the array of choices and claims is dazzling. A few people have wised up to see that the yo-yo fads ultimately lead nowhere. As a result there's been a backlash, especially against diets. There are now organisations in the US and UK which encourage women to give up the endless cycle of dieting and just accept being fat. Ironically, even those who market products have joined this backlash bandwagon. Their publicity now says, 'Don't diet, dieting is bad... except for our new miracle non-diet diet which you must try!'.

But while rejecting the whole concept of body improvement may be a relief from endless dieting and exercising, it doesn't necessarily make you feel orlook better either. Unfortunate as it is that women feel a pressure to conform to a certain image, discrimination based on appearance does exist. And there are proven medical benefits in keeping your body-fat levels low and your muscles strong.

It's All So Confusing

The fact is most people will improve their health and looks by eating and exercising properly. The problem is it's hard to know exactly *what* to do and *how* to do it. Some of the cures offered are better than others. Most will do *something*, although not necessarily what they promise or what you are seeking. But even the legitimate fitness and nutrition plans on offer can throw you into the same descending spiral if they are not practised with some forethought. The mistake so many people make over and over again is to do the wrong things to reach their goals, or to do the right things in the wrong way.

It's not that *every* book or video promoting a new exercise technique is unsafe or wrong, it's just that it is thrown at the consumer with very little explanation as to how its particular plan fits into the total scheme of body transformation. So, while the latest book of abdominal exercises may certainly *aid* in attaining a flat stomach, unless you are also following a calorie-intensive aerobic programme and are limiting the fat in your diet, it is impossible to achieve the results you expect. Without a complete understanding of how the body and exercise work, each new technique you try is inevitably doomed to fail.

Lack of Good Information

The marketplace doesn't help much, because all the books, videos and magazine articles can turn into a clotted quagmire of sound advice, quack cures, revolutionary techniques and fraudulent information. Advice is often contradictory and usually incomplete.

As a book and video reviewer for a leading fitness magazine for many years, I have read hundreds of books and watched many fitness videos. Much of what is written or presented is very basic, poorly explained, often incorrect and the authors or presenters are far from expert in the subject. Very few of them have even a basic degree in the subject they have written a book about! Often a journalist, celebrity, or underqualified specialist will be lured by the fact that miracles sell and will front a product. Even though they may have experienced real benefits from a routine and want to share the inspiration, the end product is not always reliable.

So while there are hundreds of scientific-sounding cures and answers for the multitude of 'problems', more often than not they're more marketing hype than anything else. Still the thirst for celebrity products goes on. The tide is slowly turning, however: consumers are beginning to demand advice from academically qualified nutritionists and fitness professionals. The more know-ledgeable consumers are unlikely to make the same mistakes.

What is the Answer?

Until now the solutions offered were not really solutions. If they had been, there wouldn't be so many people making the same mistakes. Everyone would be *fit*, not fat, *firm*, not flabby, *healthy*, not stressed, tired and at risk of preventable lifestyle illnesses such as heart disease.

As a fitness instructor, personal trainer and health journalist for more than 12 years, I have noticed the underlying problem – where most people go wrong and why they never achieve the goal they set out to achieve. Most people just don't know the proper facts: they have a complete misunderstanding of what to do and how to put it in action. Therefore they rarely reach their goal. In fact, the most effective approach is not something new. It's the end result of years of research by exercise scientists.

I have developed a way to help you reach your goal, which takes into account your mind *and* body. I call it the *Curves* strategy. Most exercise routines are rigid and set unrealistic goals. But, as you will discover, the fastest path to fitness isn't a straight line – it's a curve. And the curve takes into account the curves of your body and the variations in your personality.

Curves is the first book to show you how to achieve the body transformation you desire.

Do you want to improve your overall health? Lose fat? Build muscle? Increase your general stamina? Become more flexible and less tense? Once you have identified your goal, you can design a programme to achieve it. Most other fitness books on the market advocate one type of activity (such as walking, swimming or step) or present a group of exercises which focuses on a specific body part. Although many of these books claim their exercises can help achieve a variety of goals, in reality they usually can't because they don't put their exercise pro-gramme in the context of the wider realm. They don't explain how, when and why something happens. *Curves* will explain to

Jill wanted to lose weight and improve her posture. She went to several different health clubs and various classes trying to find the best type of workout, but it seemed that the various instructors all told her different, sometimes contradictory, things. One advised her not to do weights, another explained how crucial it was that she did; one told her to exercise for long periods on the aerobic machines, another told her just to walk for a short time. Stuck in a pattern, she experienced temporary weight loss but would regain it as soon as she stopped a programme.

Lesson   *Not every instructor you encounter, nor every book you read, will give you the right information. Consult several because there are a lot of uneducated people out there and it's hard to know who's right and who's wrong. Question what you're told and ask why instead of just accepting it blindly. If you receive a scientifically plausible answer and respect the qualifications of the adviser, you can probably trust the advice. Once you are sure the advice is right stick to it long enough to see if it works.*

you *how* and *why* the body burns fat, *how* to get stronger and *what to do* to decrease your risks of long-term health problems.

Curves will give you the right formula to follow and adapt to your individual characteristics.

Research has shown that there are different prescriptions for achieving various aims. There are specific programmes, each of which varies in the type, intensity, frequency and duration of exercise it recommends in order to achieve any of these goals. *Curves* will show you how to choose a programme which will take into account the many variables in your life – your individual personality, what's economically and geographically convenient, and what adjustments your body may require. You will be shown modifications to the routine to ensure that the exercises will be right for you. This knowledge will provide you with the necessary tools to assess other activities that will lead to your success.

Curves will expose some myths and give you fitness secrets.

You'll learn the truth about burning fat through exercise, how to lose fat, why it's impossible to spot reduce, the facts about cellulite, which exercise is effective and which is not, which exercise is best and how much you should do. These issues are commonly misunderstood.

Curves will help you identify all your psychological and emotional traits and take into account your practical considerations to tailor the programme to your exact needs.

Curves will help you 'input' these variables which will determine whether you stick to your programme. If you hate crowded, smelly health clubs, then taking up aerobics classes or riding the Stairmaster is not the way to ensure your success. If you live in a city, have asthma and a bad knee, then running on concrete in a polluted urban area just won't work. If you hate being alone, you might enjoy sports more than walking on a treadmill at home.

Choosing the right exercise – one that you can do easily and you enjoy – is the first step in this body transformation strategy. The second step is to learn various techniques that will help make your programme a habit, a part of your life. The *Curves* strategy will ensure that you stay motivated so that you don't give up.

As you will see when you look at the various body transformation strategies, I've catered for all fitness levels, from beginner to advanced, and the regimens are suitable for all age groups. Many of the references are to women because it's likely that more women than men will read this book but the *Curves* strategy is so individual it applies equally to men and women.

Most people – especially women – who embark on a new fitness regimen do so because they want to improve their bodies (either by losing weight or resculpting their shapes), so this forms the focus of this book. But I have also included regimens for those who just want to get healthier, increase their energy levels or relax. You'll see how different fitness programmes can affect your body in these different ways.

Curves will show you how to assess what will work for you and demonstrate how you can succeed in achieving your dream body, whatever your definition of a dream body might be.

CHAPTER 2

The Solution

What motivated you to pick up this book? Obviously you want to transform your body in some way. But how? If you don't know exactly where you're going, you'll never get there. Most people have a vague idea of what they hope to accomplish, and experiment with ways of achieving it. A few follow the right path purely by chance, but most reach a lot of dead ends.

Goals are tricky things. On the one hand you need to shoot high enough to ensure you are striving for great things. Anthony Robbins, acclaimed self-help guru and author of *Awaken the Giant Within*, says, `We must find a goal big enough and grand enough to challenge us to push beyond our limits and discover our true potential'. On the other hand, the goal can't be so unrealistic that you get lost or bored along the way – `I'm going to lose 30 pounds' or `I'm going to run a marathon'. Without some sort of interim result to keep you motivated, you'll simply never reach your goal.

But the fact is the higher your goal, the more you will achieve in attempting to attain it. Even if you don't ultimately reach this goal, you will have progressed further than you would have if you had aimed for something lower. The most effective way of achieving this big goal is to determine the steps that will lead you to it. In other words, you need to set intermediate goals to achieve the long-term ones.

Make Sure You Can Achieve It

Let's consider your overall goal. You may want to lose body fat or feel more energetic during the day. To achieve one of these aims it's essential to find out *exactly* what you need to do and then narrow your focus into easily measured, short-term goals. That way, when you achieve these lesser goals, you will be inspired to continue. If you don't achieve them, all you have to do is adjust and modify your strategy to keep you on the right path.

Let's say you want to reshape your body. This is a little vague, so let's define it further. You might decide that you want to tone up your body and lose 20 pounds (9 kg). You now have a two-part goal. This implies that you will probably have two different formulas to follow in order to achieve both.

You need to be still more specific. Identify *what parts* of your body you want to tone up so you select the right exercises. If you want to tone up your upper body and legs, you will need to do some activities or exercises which concentrate on these areas.

You also want to lose 20 pounds. Is this realistic? You may find that as your body starts to shape up, you look good without having to lose this much weight. Or 20 pounds may be too big a goal to allow a sense of accomplishment in the short term. It's hard enough to *start* exercising. So once you do, you want to make sure you feel you are achieving *something* to encourage you to continue. It's going to take quite a while to lose 20 pounds healthily. You may very well exercise solidly for one month, lose only five pounds, and then think the situation is hopeless and give up. If you give up, you'll never get the results you want. So make your goal achievable. A more realistic figure would be to shoot for five pounds. When you've reached that, you can then try for another five.

Once you've determined that you want to lose this amount of body fat, then you need to find out how to do so. In the following chapters you will discover what type of exercise will work for you.

Narrow Down Your Goal

So what is your goal?

Fitness is about self-improvement, making yourself *look* or *function* better. Ultimately it's about *feeling* better both mentally and physically. There are many results you can achieve from an exercise programme. In this book I will give you specific strategies to achieve the following four goals:

- Improving your overall health
- Increasing your energy level and stamina
- Improving your body shape through fat loss and muscle toning
- Improving your mental well-being and ability to handle stress

These are not the only benefits you will receive from exercise. The list is endless: you can improve your ability to do everyday activities such as walking up stairs; you can reduce pain caused by weak muscles around a joint; you can rehabilitate yourself from an injury; you can thwart some of the signs of ageing; you can improve your sports or athletics skills; you can learn to express your feelings through dance or aerobics. The specific changes in your body can include lower blood pressure, improved strength in your heart and lungs and a better posture.

It may be that you wish to achieve more than one of these benefits. In most cases, by working towards one, you will automatically receive some of the others. For instance, if you exercise to improve your stamina, you'll probably benefit at the same time from some improved mental alertness, a reduction in stress and possibly lose a little weight.

In order to attain these goals you need to

focus. It's not a question of simply deciding, `To reshape my body, I'm going to walk every day', and then expect, miraculously, to lose a stone. But having decided that walking is the way you're going to reach this goal, you need to determine how fast you will walk, how long you will walk and how often.

Get Specific

Exercise is specific. That means that the things you make your body do will force it to adapt to those particular stresses in specific ways. It's important to make sure that the activity or exercise you choose is actually working in the way you want it to. For example, if you stretch your muscles, your muscles will adapt by becoming more flexible. So, if you want to feel more relaxed and loose, you need to stretch, though you won't develop more endurance in your legs, heart or lungs. If you run, your legs may develop more endurance and your heart and lungs may become stronger, but you won't become more flexible.

Being fit for one activity doesn't mean you are fit for another. A perfect example is the typical aerobics class. Women seem to find aerobics a fairly easy activity to adapt to because many traditional female activities in youth, such as dancing and gymnastics, focus on co-ordination (dance) and flexibility (gymnastics) – the very components that form the focus of an aerobics class. If you have practised these movements before, you are likely to find it easier to develop these skills again.

Men, on the other hand, grew up playing sports which focused on strength, speed and power rather than co-ordination or flexibility. Therefore, stick a male athlete in an aerobics class, and he's lost! This is not to say he's not capable of developing these components of fitness, he just has to train in order to do so. In fact, many American football and basketball teams have now incorporated aerobics in their training because their traditional activities don't include much flexibility or that type of muscular endurance work. Developing this component of fitness can improve their game. Similarly, the fact that a marathon runner is very fit and can run 26 miles doesn't mean he can *swim* 26 miles. His heart and lungs may be strong from running, but his muscles will not have adapted to the movement patterns of the different activity if he has not undertaken specific training.

Keep this in mind if you think you aren't the sporty type. Your lack of co-ordination is not genetic. You just haven't been practising the right kind of skills. Or, if you think you can't do aerobics, remember it's just a matter of learning how. Once you have, you'll find that you are just as capable as anyone else.

Mary was extremely overweight and decided to hire a personal trainer. Her children were overweight too, so she thought she'd maximise the session and include them in the workout. The personal trainer arrived and sat down to assess her new client. Mary was not interested in the preliminaries and asked if they could just work out. So the trainer started a gentle stretch and conditioning session. With five kids of varying ages trying to follow, it became more of a kindergarten than a workout. Mary decided exercise wasn't for her and never called the trainer again.

Lesson *If you have been turned off exercise, stop and reconsider. Was it the actual exercise or the conditions surrounding it? Was your goal realistic? Did you approach it in the right way? The Curves strategy will help you define a practical, achievable programme.*

Do the Right Thing

There is a wide variety of activities you can do to achieve one of the four goals (health, energy, body reshaping and serenity). Muscles move in different ways, in different combinations and at different speeds and intensities. To reach your goal, you need to determine the right exercise prescription that will get you there.

It may be that you don't need to do as much as you think. Or you may need to do more, or something different. So many people waste time following the wrong programme, or doing the right programme in the wrong way. Perhaps the biggest misconception most people have is the actual amount and type of exercise they need to do.

Many women believe that by following the type of exercise done in Callanetics they will reshape their bodies and lose unwanted inches. This method uses isometric exercise, which simply means squeezing your muscles. This has a certain appeal because it takes very little effort or movement to focus on a muscle and squeeze. But it also uses very little energy. Losing fat, weight and inches requires that you use a large amount of energy so that your body's fat stores will get used up. So, according to all physiological principles, it would be difficult to lose fat with this method.

Even reshaping the body and firming the muscles usually requires a muscle to move throughout its full range of motion and against considerable resistance. When you squeeze a muscle you strengthen a small portion, but not all of it. A recent study at the University of Westminster sought to determine whether or not the claims made in the original Callanetics products were true. The researchers found no significant differences in body weight, body fat, body measurements, or muscular strength and endurance after participants completed ten hours of the programme. Although isometric exercise may *feel* as if it's working because doing the exercises causes a muscle-burning sensation, the method may actually be ineffective.

Fitness Goals

Do You Want To:

Improve the efficiency of your body?

Do you want to become more flexible, release tension in your shoulders and back, improve your posture, or feel less fatigued after climbing stairs? Depending on what you wish to improve, you'll need to do the right exercises to achieve it. Flexibility improvements require slow stretching exercises working towards moving each joint progressively through greater ranges of motion. If you want to improve your posture, performing specific exercises for muscles in your back and shoulders and also stretching the muscles in your back, chest and thighs will help.

Reduce pain or get fit after an illness?

Do you have a weak lower back, an injured shoulder or knee, or heart disease? You'll need to consult a qualified physiotherapist for specific advice on which muscles or physiological systems to strengthen.

Improve the way you handle stress?

To relax or have a healthy outlet for work or personal stress, many types of exercise, including walking and yoga, can help.

Improve your mental well-being?

Do you want to be able to meditate, distance yourself from your problems, relax and feel a sense of inner peace? There is much research to show that you can achieve immediate mental benefits such as improved self-esteem and decreased anxiety and depression from almost any type of exercise, regardless of how fit you are.

Improve your sports skills?

To run a marathon, improve your tennis serve, or swim five days a week, you'll need to get some help from the relevant professional. But improving your fitness level by *basic* activities can also improve your performance in any sport.

Lose weight and/or body fat?

You will find later in this book the most effective ways to do this and discover which methods are almost a complete waste of time.

Reshape your body?

Muscle-conditioning exercises will firm up different areas of your body or resculpt your physique. Depending on whether you just want to firm up, or also need to lose weight in order to gain muscle definition, there are specific programmes to follow.

Improve your overall health?

If you are concerned for your long-term welfare and want to decrease your risks of heart problems and other diseases and improve the *quality* of your life as you age, small regular amounts of low-intensity activity can help. As well as keeping your body healthy and strong, exercise can help your co-ordination and even help maintain mental sharpness which decreases with age.

What Will Work For You?

The more unfit you are, the more results you will see merely by starting to move again. In such cases it's important to start doing *something*. If your body has got out of the habit of moving, almost any activity you do is likely to produce noticeable results. You need to be as specific as you can in setting your goals, but the main thing is to start.

The more fit you are and the smaller the changes you seek (perhaps losing ten pounds instead of fifty), the more important it is for you to be very specific and consistent.

If you just want to improve your general health or feel better mentally, simple stretching, occasional walks or cycling may be enough. But in small doses these activities won't be effective if you want significantly to change the way you look. Weight loss and muscle definition require a reasonable amount of time (a few months) and a larger amount of exercise than most people expect. As you learn in the next few chapters how your body operates, you will understand why this is so. See Chart One on p.000 for general descriptions of what you need to do to achieve various fitness goals.

Examine Your Motives

If you would like to lose weight or change your body shape, consider *why* you want to do this. You probably want to look better and therefore feel more self-confident. The fact is, unless you feel good *regardless* of whether you are five pounds overweight, you won't necessarily feel any better by losing weight. If you do, it will only be temporary. There is no guarantee that if you become beautiful and slim life will be so much more enjoyable and you will be more confident and satisfied. *The truth is, there is no miracle diet or exercise plan that will give you freedom from self-doubt and insecurity.* In fact, many bestselling diets, fitness techniques and beauty products thrive on making you feel insecure, hence the increase in eating disorders such as anorexia and bulimia. Until you are aware of this, you can easily fall victim to self-destructive motives. So stand back and put the whole thing into perspective.

The Forces Against You

The beauty industry thrives on encouraging a woman's need to change her face, body and image. It targets women's insecurities over what is perceived to be their physical abnormalities. Anything that could be a physical `problem' is marketed as such and its victims sold the cure. The cult of the supermodel perpetuates this insidious obsession. Whether Linda, Cindy, Naomi or Claudia have talent or intellect is irrelevant, they are revered only for the way they look.

But for many who idolise the ideal, the look is unattainable. The images we see in glossy magazines not only represent a tiny percentage of women genetically inclined to look that way but are often distorted through airbrushing – entire body parts can be reshaped in photos by special computer technology. Lighting, make-up, camera angles and plastic surgery all contribute to the illusion. Ordinary women just don't stand a chance of looking the way the pictures touting their products suggest they can. So the woman trying to look this good will be trying for ever.

Trapped by Self-Consciousness

At the very least a woman is trapped in a life of self-criticism. By having standards that can never be attained – thin enough thighs, white enough teeth – a woman will feel eternally inadequate. If she's not constantly doing something, she feels guilty about it: or she is saying to herself, `Oh, I shouldn't have eaten that chocolate cake'. This cycle of self-reproach makes women who succumb to it a willing target for the next miracle gimmick that comes along offering to solve their problems.

Enough is Enough

At some point enough is enough. The answer is not to give up all attempts to improve your looks because the undeniable fact is, prejudice does exist and you just might miss out on important opportunities. Studies have shown that attractive people get better jobs and are better paid. To a certain extent you have to play the game. So, yes, get fit and firm up your body, but don't let it turn into an obsession. Calculate the amount of time you spend getting dressed or refining your looks: if you spend more than seven hours a week, consider whether that time might be better spent doing something else. Don't let your appearance rule your life: accept yourself as you are; concentrate on building strengths on the inside, not just the outside; be realistic about your goals.

Later in the book, you will find four general fitness Body Transformation Curves. By following these you can improve your health, increase your energy levels, reduce body fat and reshape your body, and handle stress. These curves are based on guidelines set by the international governing body of fitness, the American College of Sports Medicine.

The next few chapters will teach you how your body works. Once you have a basic understanding of how physical changes take place, you'll recognise the path you need to take. But, because everyone is different, you'll also pinpoint some of the personal adaptations you'll need to make to tailor the programme to suit your exact requirements.

CHAPTER 3

The Metabolic Miracle

The human body is a miraculous thing. Not many people truly appreciate it. It wasn't chance that let us scale up the evolutionary ladder. Our bodies are able to adapt to tackle the stresses that life presents. Historically this meant different changes for different situations. If a man had to walk hours during a hunt for food, his body developed the ability to do this: his feet developed callouses, his muscles gained endurance, his body learned to use its energy stores most efficiently. If a bacteria or virus invaded his system, he developed antibodies which would kill them, in some cases making him immune from further attacks.

To become fit for survival, our biggest coup was developing the ability to avoid starvation by storing supplies of energy, usually in the form of fat. If you are interested in losing weight or body fat, the next three chapters will explain how the energy you eat and the energy you use through exercise affect your body.

YOUR METABOLISM

Where Do I Get Energy?

Your energy comes from three food sources: carbohydrates, protein and fat. So when you eat fat, for instance, it is stored throughout the body and used later for energy. Carbohydrates are stored mostly in your muscles. Protein is stored in your hair, skin and nails. Protein is rarely used for energy but acts as a back-up when your fat and carbohydrate stores are depleted. Only

someone ill or starving, such as an anorexic, will get energy from protein.

Think of the energy sources as items you use at home. Carbohydrates are the most accessible – you might put them on a shelf by your desk for easy reach when you need them. Fat requires more effort to get used up – it might be something you keep in a closet. Protein would be stored in the attic because it's only needed for energy under special circumstances.

How Much Energy Does the Body Use?

Fat, carbohydrates and protein are measured according to how much heat, or calories, they produce. To meet your daily physical demands you will burn both fat and carbohydrate calories. Fat is our main energy source because it is abundant everywhere in the body while carbohydrates and protein are stored in very limited supplies. We have hundreds of thousands of fat calories stored to ensure the smooth functioning of our bodies. The number of calories we use is determined by two factors: basic metabolism and additional activity.

Your basic metabolism is the minimum amount of energy your body needs in a resting state to maintain basic life processes such as cell growth and renewal, digestion, sleep and thinking. Although it is difficult to measure without laboratory equipment, it can be estimated that a 27-year-old woman who is 5 feet 6 inches (1.7 m) tall and weighs 9 stone 10 pounds (61.7 kg) might need to consume at least 1500 calories per day. So her basic metabolic rate is said to be about 1500 calories. If she eats more than this she will gain weight. If she eats less she will lose weight.

You can increase the amount of calories you use each day by the amount of activity and exercise you do. If you exercise vigorously for an hour you might use 600 calories. Therefore you would need to eat an additional 600 calories worth of food in order to maintain your current weight. If you didn't consume these extra calories, then you would start to lose weight.

How Can I Increase My Metabolism?

Your metabolism is fairly static and depends mainly on your height and weight. In general, the heavier a person, the more calories they will burn since it takes more energy to move more weight. If your metabolism is high you may find that you can eat a lot without seeming to gain any weight. On the other hand, if it's slow you may find it easy to gain weight and difficult to lose it.

Exercise may help increase your metabolism so that you burn up calories more quickly. Certainly, *while* you are exercising you increase your metabolism, but there is little evidence to show that you can raise your *overall* metabolic rate. After periods of very intense exercise you raise your metabolic rate slightly for a few hours. This is a temporary boost, though the accumulated calorie loss may still aid in weight loss over a period of time.

However, the amount of muscle and fat you have and how fit you are will also determine how many calories you burn. More muscle means more metabolically active, calorie-burning tissue. *The more muscle you have, the more calories your body will use throughout the day, even when resting.* Since men have more muscle mass and are heavier than women, they usually have a higher metabolic rate.

The fitter you are, the more fuel-efficient your body becomes. You can last longer before becoming fatigued and therefore burn more calories. Many athletes are able to eat a lot without gaining weight. Most likely this is due to the large amounts of activity they do, the increased muscle mass in their bodies, and the increased efficiency of their muscles. *The more active you are, the more active is your metabolism.*

As you age, your metabolism slows down. Whether this is due to ageing or simply the tendency to decrease activity levels (which results in more fat and less muscle) is debatable. It is particularly important, however, to stay active as you grow older.

How Does Dieting Affect My Metabolism?

A reduction in the number of calories you eat makes your metabolism slow down. It's the body's way of preserving energy. A slower metabolism is a normal response to the weight being lost. The lower your weight, the less energy your body needs.

Yo-yo dieting or drastic eating patterns which cause your weight to fluctuate and a loss of muscle mass may also lower your metabolism, which is why these are not healthy or effective ways to lose weight. Although dieting causes your metabolism to slow down, if you are also exercising your metabolism may, in the long term, return to normal levels.

HOW TO LOSE WEIGHT

Through the ages fat has been our greatest tool for survival. Ironically, we're now trying to beat it into submission. But, while 20th-century man has waged war against it, the fat is fighting back: fat is damned hard to lose. The irony is that some people have too much of it and can't seem to get rid of it, while others stay slim no matter what they eat. The problem lies not in the body, but in the mind. We step on the scales and lament when the needle inches its way up when, in fact, we should be jubilant at building up our fat stores. Instead, the body gets starved and battered, just for doing what it does best.

But body fat *can* be decreased – it's just a matter of understanding the rules. Most fitness experts agree that the formula is straightforward: if you eat more calories than you use, you will gain weight; if you use more calories than you eat, you will lose weight. In an ideal world this formula would work, but for many it's not that simple.

First, many people who want to lose weight actually want to lose fat. Without realising this, they judge the success of the diet or exercise plan by the reading on the bathroom scales, which cannot accurately measure fat loss. *Weight loss and fat loss are not the same.*

Since up to 60 per cent of our body weight is water, you can lose ˋwater weight' almost immediately. Going on a crash diet (fewer than 1200 calories) means your body is not getting enough energy from the food you eat. So it is forced to use up the available carbohydrates for energy. When carbohydrates are broken down, a by-product of the process is water. Therefore when excess carbohydrates are burnt, water is excreted from the body, causing weight loss. The same process occurs during very vigorous exercise. In addition tosweating, you may notice that you have to use the toilet immediately after a high-intensity session. You can lose pounds of water quickly, but this is not what we want to achieve.

Why Weight Loss Can Be Deceiving

There are several problems with losing ˋwater weight'. First, since very little (if any) fat is lost, you cannot drastically change your body shape, which is what you really want. Second, water is necessary for the proper functioning of your body. You can feel tired and sick unless you keep yourself well hydrated. Third, if you have lost ˋwater weight', the next time you eat or drink the fluids will be replaced (most foods contain water) and the weight regained. *Quick weight loss is not permanent.* It can account for the wild fluctuations from regular dieters who lose ten pounds one week and gain ten pounds the next.

In addition, if the weight loss is too drastic, you may lose not only water but vital lean tissues. Your metabolism will slow down to conserve energy. There is also an increase in an enzyme which causes fat to be stored – very counterproductive if you're trying to lose fat. Over a period of time, energy may even be taken from protein stores in the body (including the hair and skin). Since the brain needs a form of carbohydrate to operate, if these stores are depleted, your mental functions could be impaired. All of these changes make weight gain more likely and weight loss much more difficult.

Several studies have indicated that combining exercise with a weight-loss diet can prevent the loss of lean muscle tissue and thwart the lowering ofmetabolic rate. Assuming the calorie reduction is modest, this method appears to work.

Kelly was a sucker for any new diet, beauty treatment or exercise technique. She was also constantly battling with a slight weight problem. Her usual method of losing weight in time for a special event was fasting. Although she'd been told that fasting ultimately messed up her metabolism even more, she didn't really believe it. She got the immediate weight-loss result she needed, *when* she needed it. The problem is the weight loss never lasted. For the past ten years Kelly had yo-yoed.

Lesson *There's no reason to think that Kelly's yo-yo syndrome will ever stop. In fact, there is evidence to suggest that her weight will increase regularly over the next few decades to combat the stresses being put on her body. Rather than put her body through such drastic extremes, she would do better to adopt a sensible, stable plan of regular exercise and calorie maintenance.*

But if you over-exercise you may experience the same risks. Excessive exercise without eating enough calories may cause the same slower metabolic changes that crash dieting induces because the body still detects a drastic calorific reduction. An obsessive exerciser may find that he or she can exercise *less* and experience the same or more benefits in fitness and weight loss.

The key to successful weight loss is to incorporate moderate dieting with moderate exercise.

How Do I Lose Body Fat?

Fat loss can greatly affect the way you look, although it does not necessarily mean a change of actual body weight. If the fat loss is achieved slowly over a period of time (especially through exercise), it is likely that there will be a gradual change in your muscle-to-fat ratio. You will gain muscle and lose fat, resulting in little change in actual pounds but a significant difference in your appearance.

Fat loss can result in a loss of body weight if more fat is lost than muscle tissue gained. *One pound of fat is equivalent to about 3500 calories so 3500 calories worth of exercise could cause one pound (0.5 kg) of fat loss.* Depending upon the individual, it might take about nine hours of walking or six hours of running *over a period of time* to burn up this number of calories. Since this is a slower progression to a lower body weight, the body is able to adapt without going into a protective response and the weight loss is more likely to be permanent.

The international governing body of exercise, the American College of Sports Medicine (ACSM), advocates fat loss through a slight reduction in food (eating no fewer than 1200 calories per day) and by expending a greater number of calories. *For permanent weight loss, eat a little less and exercise a little more for the rest of your life.* The call to exercise is universally acknowledged: it's the *type* of exercise – walking, swimming, weights, aerobics, anaerobics, and so on – which has been the subject of much misunderstanding.

HOW TO BURN FAT THROUGH EXERCISE

All the cells in our body need energy. As mentioned earlier in this chapter, the two main sources of energy are fat and carbohydrates. Fat requires oxygen in order to be broken down for fuel: this process is known as aerobic metabolism. Carbohydrates do not require oxygen in order to be broken down and used: this is anaerobic metabolism.

Most cells, like those in the heart, lungs and brain, need oxygen in order to produce energy. But muscle cells are able to produce energy even when oxygen molecules are not present. This is useful when you need immediate or intense amounts of energy. If your oxygen intake (the amount you breathe) cannot increase fast enough for more fat to be broken down, the muscles can break down another substance for fuel – carbohydrates.

Throughout the day we rely primarily on aerobic metabolism, so even as you sit here reading you are burning fat! Of course the intensity at which you are sitting requires very little energy, so you are not burning very much fat. If you were to get up and dance, your energy would increase and you would burn more calories.

Because the act of getting up suddenly requires immediate energy, your body shifts to anaerobic metabolism to supply it with some quick energy. If you were to start dancing moderately, your body would switch back to the more efficient aerobic metabolism. Aerobic exercise burns more fat. Walking, running, aerobic dance, cycling, swimming and other endurance activities can be aerobic, but not always.

Working Out Very Hard

The important factor is not the activity, but the intensity at which it is performed. In other words, if the amount of energy you need and the amount of fat your body is able to produce are similar, the activity will be aerobic, in other words, use more fat. If you require more energy than your body can produce aerobically, the activity will rely on quick energy-supplying carbohydrates for its fuel.

Aerobic exercise performed at low to medium intensity relies mostly on fat to fuel the movement. Since fat is in plentiful supply, this type of metabolism is endurance-oriented; you have more energy available so you can last longer. But the harder you work, the more your body draws on carbohydrates to meet its increasing energy demands. If you work out too hard and your intensity is too high, your carbohydrate levels deplete significantly, and your work level then has to drop if your body is to revert to use of fats. That's why you can easily walk for 30 minutes, but not sprint for 30 minutes. *So if you run slowly you may burn more fat. If you run hard and fast you may burn more carbohydrates.* Before you conclude that you should only run slowly, read on.

When you exercise, your fitness level will also determine which fuel is favoured. The less fit you are, even an aerobic activity such as walking can be anaerobic. A trained person will have a greater fat-burning capacity than an unfit person because the fit person will have a more efficient metabolism and an increased sensitivity in his or her muscles, which helps to metabolise fat. Some ultramarathoners (those who participate in runs lasting up to 24 hours) can reach a point where they are burning 95 per cent fat to fuel theirmovements. *As the body becomes fitter, it becomes more efficient and learns to favour fat. The fitter you are the greater the possibility that your body will be able to use fat even during high-intensity exercise.*

Muscle-conditioning exercises, on the other hand, do not use fat for fuel. The majority of energy is produced from carbohydrates. Exercises such as calisthenics (sit-ups, push-ups, leg lifts) and weight training, where you focus intensely on one or two particular muscle groups and work them to the point of fatigue, *can* strengthen your muscles, but they will not use body fat for fuel.

The Fat-Burning Myth

Those who work out to lose weight or improve their body shape often assume they should do aerobic exercise to burn fat. Exercise done at a low intensity, such as walking, is often touted as being more fat-burning than other high-intensity activities. While, in theory, these claims may be true, whether increased fat burning will result in actual weight loss is dependent upon several variables, including the total *calories* burned (which includes both fat and carbohydrate calories) and the total *fat calories* burned.

For example, at rest (i.e. doing nothing) you may burn up to 60 per cent fat – the remaining 40 per cent is primarily carbohydrate. When you enter the initial phases of intense exercise, the ratio changes. You may now burn only 30 per cent fat because your body is using quick-energy carbohydrates. Once the exercise is established, the body switches back to using a higher percentage of fat (up to 75 per cent) to fuel the movement. *In this low-intensity aerobic phase of exercise, a higher percentage of fat is being used for energy. But ifyou are not working out for a very long period you may still burn more total calories and, therefore, more fat calories working out harder.*

High-Intensity vs. Low-Intensity Exercise

Because working at a lower intensity requires less quick energy, more fat is burned than during high-intensity activity. This, though, is where the misinterpretation might be made. Even though a higher percentage of fat is used, since you are working at a lower intensity you are burning fewer calories overall. Even though a *higher percentage* of fat is being used, a *lower total amount* of fat is lost. *Working out at a very low intensity in order to burn fat is the fat-burning myth. You may actually be worse off in terms of weight loss because you are burning fewer calories overall.* If you do work at a low intensity you need to increase the time spent exercising in order to burn more calories.

Let's say you have 30 minutes to work out. If you were to walk, you would burn fewer calories than if you were to run. To burn the same amount of calories as you would when running, you would need to walk for an extra 15 or 20 minutes. *So if you are exercising for 30 minutes, you will burn more total fat calories working at a higher, rather than a lower intensity.* Working out at higher intensities may cause you to burn a *lower percentage* of fat, but since you will be using more calories in total, you will still be using more fat calories. Since weight loss is considered to be most effective when the largest number of calories are used, it is impossible to lose *more* weight from a lower-intensity exercise programme unless you exercise for longer periods of time.

Low-intensity exercise can burn a significant number of calories *over a period of time.* Aerobic activities allow you to last longer, therefore using up more calories. *Many people who cannot physically handle high-intensity exercise can experience the same results by doing low-intensity workouts.* This is a perfectly acceptable approach, especially if you're not the type that likes to sweat or push yourself too hard. Just be patient as the results take a little longer.

Can I Lose Weight From Exercise Alone?

Despite many claims of miraculous weight loss from a variety of exercise regimes, there are few studies that show you can lose a significant amount of weight from moderate exercise alone. The immediate effects of exercise are limited because small doses of exercise burn relatively small numbers of calories. You might burn 300 calories in a half-hour brisk walk, but then eat more than 1000 calories in a fast-food meal of a hamburger, french fries and soft drink.

The *cumulative* effects of exercise can make a difference, however. Small numbers of calories used will add up to pounds lost, even though it may take months. If you are exercising vigorously at a very high intensity over a long period of time you may be able to burn enough calories to effect a sizeable body change in a relatively short period of time (three or more months). But if the exercise intensity has been, or is, too high the body produces lactic acid which inhibits fat breakdown making it much harder to burn fat. Most people do not find it easy to stick to an intense programme, so just work at the level that feels most comfortable for you. The key to success is not how many calories you burn during one session but how many you can use over a period of time.

Myth

You can use specific exercises to spot reduce

False. To reduce fat from your body you must decrease your fat stores. To decrease fat you must burn calories. But there is no evidence to prove that you can control which of the fat stores are used. No matter how many leg lifts or stomach exercises you do, they will probably not cause any inch loss from these areas. In fact, if you use enough resistance you may even gain inches of muscle mass. Calorie-burning endurance exercise like walking and running will help you lose fat from all over the body, including these areas. But you should do the specific muscle-conditioning exercises in addition because there is some evidence that the more muscle fibre you have, the more energy you use. Therefore, resistance exercises are recommended, but they must be done in conjunction with calorie-intensive activities.

Weight Loss From Exercise and Diet

Exercise can greatly enhance the success of a weight-loss diet. One study found that subjects who combined endurance exercise with weight training while on a diet lost an average of 32 per cent more weight than those who dieted without taking exercise.

Since the bigger problem lies not in losing the weight but in keeping it off, exercise is a crucial ingredient for maintaining weight loss over a period of time.

Why Doesn't Anything Seem to Work for Me?

Despite valiant efforts, you may still find it difficult to lose weight or fat. Here are some of the reasons why.

- **Not using enough calories** Most common is that you may simply not be using up enough calories. Working out once or twice a week at a low intensity may be enough to achieve or maintain health benefits but not enough to achieve weight loss. Exercising four or five days a week at moderate intensity/medium duration *or* low intensity/long duration will probably be more effective. In addition, increasing the energy you use in day-to-day activities can add up too: walk instead of taking the bus; use the stairs instead of the lift.

- **Giving up** Commitment is the key to weight loss. Exercise should be continued on a long-term basis. Many people give up before they have had a chance to see results. It will take as long to lose it as it did to gain it.

- **Overeating** You may be miscalculating the number of calories you eat either by underestimating your portions or by neglecting to include the nibbling along the way. Try eating smaller portions rather than starving yourself.

- **What you inherit** There is some evidence that your body has a set point where it keeps weight regulated at a particular level. It can be difficult to move beyond this level.

Research has also shown that heredity may predispose some to have a higher number of fat cells. The body is not a piece of clay: there are certain genetic factors which you may not be able to alter.

Specific patterns of body-fat distribution are also genetic. Lower-body fat seems to be more resilient, possibly for energy storage during childbearing. However, upper-body fat, especially in the abdominal area, seems to indicate a higher risk of heart disease. There is also some evidence that the type of muscle fibre you have may affect your fat-burning ability. Some people are natural fat burners and those with another type of muscle fibre are natural carbohydrate burners.

- **Mindset** If you don't *believe* it will happen, the chances are, it won't. Essentially, you can give two physiologically identical people the same diet and exercise plan and end up with different results. It's important to have the right attitude and mindset to be successful with your diet and exercise regimen.

How Do I Gain Weight?

For obvious health reasons, gaining too much fat is not the best way to gain weight. Building more muscle mass is. You don't have to eat a great deal more, just change the proportions of what you eat. Aim for a high-carbohydrate diet.

The next step is increasing your muscle mass. An intensive, regular strength training programme should help put on weight. Perhaps the best focus for the programme should be on developing as much muscle bulk as possible. This will give a skinny person the illusion of being much bigger.

Doing three sets of 8-12 repetitions of exercises using fairly heavy weights is the most effective way to build bulk.

Slowing down an active lifestyle may help conserve energy as well. Against all the usual advice, try taking the lift instead instead of walking upstairs. As long as you are helping your overall health through regular exercise, you can try to avoid burning too many extra calories.

CHAPTER 4

Muscles

You may not think you want muscles. But if you want curves, you want muscles. Muscles in women are very rarely the masculine, vein-popping bulges of the average body builder which is actually a very difficult look to achieve. As they are the support system of your skeleton, well-developed muscles will give you superb posture and improve your overall body shape drastically. Finely tuned muscles mean you will also move with more grace and precision.

A muscle cell is shaped like a long cylinder which runs the length of the muscle and is therefore called a muscle fibre. A group of muscle fibres are wrapped in a membrane to form a muscle bundle. Many muscle bundles are enclosed in another membrane to form the muscle. Each muscle is responsible for the specific action of a bone or group of bones. The human body resembles a marionette with muscles acting as pulleys and bones acting as levers. Many muscles may work together when you perform a particular movement.

How Do My Muscles Become Stronger?

When you work a muscle just beyond what it is used to, it is forced to work extra hard to overcome the load. In doing so, the fibres break down, causing tiny microtears. Within approximately 48 hours of rest they heal and grow stronger by increasing their amount of muscle proteins. Your tendons (fibres connecting muscle to bone), ligaments (fibres connecting bones) and bones will also become stronger when exposed to resistance. This means your joint will be much more stable.

Each individual fibre contains proteins which are continually being made and broken down in a process know as turnover. It has been estimated that about 25 per cent of the total protein in a muscle is in a state of turnover at any one time. If strength in a muscle stays the same it's because the breakdown rate equals that of the build-up.

During the initial stages of a resistance programme the muscle gets stronger by learning how to operate more efficiently. There are improvements in the way the muscles co-ordinate with the nerves and in the number of muscle fibres used during a given movement. Later, the addition of more protein into the fibres accounts for thicker, stronger muscles.

Myth

Leg lifts will produce skinny legs

False. Physiologists have found that the fuel source used in calisthenic (anaerobic) exercise is glycogen (carbohydrates) and not fat (as in aerobic exercise). For this reason, even 1000 repetitions will not burn much fat from the thigh. However, these exercises will firm and strengthen the muscles providing greater support for the knees and hips.

What is the Difference Between Muscle Strength and Muscle Endurance?

When a muscle is challenged, it adapts in several different ways. If your body is exposed to external resistance, your muscles can adapt by growing stronger, developing more staying power, or acquiring the ability to move more efficiently. The type of resistance plan you follow will determine which of the adaptations will occur.

Muscle *strength* refers to the amount of force a muscle can produce – how much weight you can lift, for instance. Lifting progressively heavier weights will help you develop strength.

Muscle *endurance* refers to the ability of a muscle to contract repeatedly over a period of time. So doing exercises in which you focus on maintaining the work for longer will help you develop endurance. Many activities require that you develop a certain amount of staying power in order to participate. If you decide to cycle long distances, for example, your thighs and buttocks must be able to last as well as your heart and lungs.

Any resistance-training programme will develop both strength and endurance, but the amount of weight you lift and the number of repetitions you do will determine which benefit you develop more. The general rule is to use heavier weights with lower repetitions to build strength and to use lighter weights with higher repetitions to build endurance.

Muscle *power* is the ability to generate a large amount of force quickly. This type of muscular adaptation is more sports related. Athletes who jump or execute powerful movements will train to develop this skill.

Why Should I Do Specific Muscle Conditioning?

It used to be that resistance training to condition the muscles was seen as mostly an aesthetic pursuit – to achieve the sculpted 'body beautiful'. Endurance exercise such as walking or cycling was considered more important because it strengthened the heart and lungs and elicited various beneficial internal changes in the body.

Recently, however, the consensus is that training for muscular strength and endurance is as important as other types of exercise. Not only will you increase the stability of your joints and other skeletal structures, which can prevent or help combat weakness in the body (including the lower back), you can also thwart the loss of muscle that comes with age. Resistance and weight-bearing exercise is crucial in maintaining bone strength and in providing protection from injury. Of course it will also help you lose weight and improve the way you look.

How Do I Get Better Muscle Tone and Definition?

Tone and *definition* are the physical characteristics a muscle will have as a result of developing strength, endurance and/or power. Tone is how tight, or firm the muscle is. Definition is how sculpted it looks.

You can develop a certain amount of tone by doing any type of exercise. The firmer you want to be, however, the more you need to do specific exercises with weights or elastic bands. General guidelines for resistance training are to use weights which are heavy enough so that your muscles feelfatigued after the first 8-12 repetitions. If they don't, you need to use more resistance. If you cannot complete eight you need to use less.

Muscle definition is harder to achieve because it depends on your body-fat levels. The more lean you are and the less fat you have, the more sculpted or 'cut' your muscles will appear because you have less fat to fill out the curves of your muscles in your body. Professional body-builders achieve the cut, sculpted look not only by building muscle bulk, but also by reducing their body fat to very low levels. Combining calorie-burning exercise such as walking, aerobics, or cycling with your weight training will help you look more defined.

I Had Muscle Tone When I Was Younger, But Now It's All Turned to Fat

Contrary to popular belief, a muscle will not turn into fat. Muscle tissue may be lost and fat tissue may be increased, but one will not turn into the other. If a muscle is unused for a period – while in a plaster cast, for example – the breakdown of muscle tissue exceeds the build-up and the muscle will atrophy, or waste away. As you become more inactive, your fat levels usually increase due to excess calories being stored.

If you have embarked on a weight-lifting programme but then stop the regular training, any gains you have made in performance and strength will be noticeably lost three to four weeks after stopping. The lack of work is perceived as a lack of demand, so the ability declines. This is not to say that you have to lift weights three times a week for the rest of your life. Once you reach a desired level, to maintain it, studies suggest that all you need to do is lift once or twice per week.

How Can I Avoid Bulking Up Too Much?

How bulky your muscles look depends on several factors. These include:

- **Genetics** The composition of muscles varies from one individual to another. Some people may be born with more muscle cells than others. Also, skeletal structure plays a major role in determining how muscular a person looks. A very tall, lean man with long bones will find it difficult to get extremely bulky. Likewise, a shorter, stockier man may find he bulks up quite easily.

There are several types of muscle fibres. Although most people have approximately equal amounts of each type, some muscles and some people may have slightly higher proportions of one than another. This may make them appear more or less bulky.

- **Type of training** The type of resistance and training affects how big your muscles get. Lifting heavier weights results in more bulk. But heavy means anything from 20 pounds (9 kg), not the light weights of 1-12 pounds (0.5-5.4 kg) used by most women.

- **Sex** Women tend to have less muscle mass (especially in the upper body) and less testosterone, so it is impossible to look like a body builder unless you are doing serious training with heavy weights and taking steroids or other muscle-building substances.

What Type of Exercise Will Make My Muscles Long and Lean?

Long, slim muscles are considered the ideal. But creating that shape is not as simple as doing a few 'lengthening' exercises. Dancers' bodies are often used as a standard. But dancers' limbs are not necessarily a product of the moves they do. More likely it's the way they do them and their genetic make-up.

Studies have shown that resistance train-ing done *slowly* develops more muscle mass, and dancers tend to move through resistance with greater speed. It may be that this type of movement will stimulate the muscles enough to keep them growing stronger without increasing visible bulk. But it's a myth to believe that, if you take up ballet, you can significantly change the way your body looks. You can control your muscle tone and bulk up to a point, but then other factors enter into the equation.

Not all dancers have skinny legs. If you went to a ballet company rehearsal you would find all types of body shapes. But the leading companies tend to choose dancers who look long and thin – especially for leading roles and won't accept a dancer unless he or she has thin, long limbs. At these auditions they measure the dancers, look at their parents and insist you look like an ostrich before you even get a part.

Other potentially harmful factors can mould a dancer into the required shape. With practice sessions of eight to ten hours a day, there is often little time to eat enough or eat at all. It would be hard for anyone to develop much muscle or gain any weight if they were burning several thousand calories a day and eating little food. Several studies have shown that most dancers are protein-deficient. If you picture the classic ballet dancer, she has a wasted upper body and torso because any protein she gets is shifted to maintain her lower body musculature: in effect many dancers are cannibalising themselves. They can end up with injuries that never heal and often with anorexia.

Many women are attracted to dance and shun weight training for fear of getting too big. If you are worried, stick to endurance activities and keep the resistance low when using weights or doing other powerful movements, such as cycling or stepping.

Tom had always been tall and thin. He wanted to get a more muscular body so he started going to the gym to use the stationery bike and the Stairmaster and to lift free weights. He remained scrawny. After a month he didn't see a difference so he stopped.

Lesson *To build muscle mass Tom would have had to stick to a progressive weight-lifting programme. He gave up too soon and did not keep challenging his muscles to grow.*

Will Resistance Training Help Me Lose Weight?

Studies have shown that doing resistance training and endurance training together is better because as you decrease your fat stores your body will become firmer too.

What Kind of Resistance Can I Use?

The three main types of resistance equipment available are weight machines (as you would see in the gym), free weights (dumbbells and weighted bars) and elastic bands.

- **Weight machines** require you to push or pull a weight stack attached to a pulley or chain. Some machines have a form of hydraulics to provide resistance. If you are a beginner, machines are the best since they have a designated seat and handles. These automatically put you in the proper position to perform an exercise. Since the weight is held away from your body, there is less risk of it dropping on you. But the fixed position of each piece of equipment means that the choice of positions in which you can work a muscle is somewhat limited.

- **Free weights** can give you a more flexible workout. You can work a muscle more thoroughly because you can perform the same exercise in a variety of planes. Most exercises with weights isolate a particular muscle and work it alone before working another muscle. With free weights you can isolate muscles *or* work them in groups. This is especially useful in training for sports which require several muscles to co-ordinate together to perform a skill such as simulating a tennis serve or making a swimming motion.

  In order to lift free weights properly you need control and co-ordination. You also need proper instruction to show you how to do the exercises correctly.

• **Elastic bands** may look flimsy, but several studies have shown they can give your muscles an effective strength-training workout. These items were used initially by physiotherapists as an inexpensive method of rehabilitation that the patient could continue to use at home. Now their use is widespread in fitness classes.

Elastic bands and tubes operate on the principle that the elastic has a certain amount of tension. To stretch the band, your muscle must exert increasing levels of force to overcome the resistance. The bands usually come in different strengths.

The more flexible they are, the less resistance on your muscles.

Bands can have limitations: they are often awkward to grip, though now some come with handles; if they are too tight, they may cause you to squeeze your muscle without moving it, an ineffective way to train.

If you are hypertensive, check with your doctor before beginning a resistance training programme. Since the exertion caused by lifting weights or stretching bands increases your blood pressure, it is best to stick to very low resistances.

Myth

Cellulite is a build-up of toxic wastes in your body

False. The beautician Nicole Ronsard popularised the idea of cellulite in *Cellulite: Those Lumps, Bumps and Bulges You Couldn't Lose Before*, published in 1973. This led to a spate of books, products and treatments offering a cure. The premise was that those dimples on your hips and thighs were cellulite, a medical imbalance predominantly in female bodies. What had previously been known as just plain fat was now apparently the build-up of toxic water caused by poor circulation and a sluggish lymphatic system. This has worried so many women that any cellulite book offering a remedy is guaranteed to sell. But a host of medical and physiological experts have dismissed the claims about this mysterious ingredient of women's thighs.

The consensus is that these dimples are just plain fat. True, there are different fat cell compositions – the dimples develop on women's hips, thighs and buttocks for both genetic and sex-related reasons. It is visible because it is directly beneath the skin rather than stored deeper in the body. Lower-body fat, in particular, is hormonal and serves as a back-up energy store for pregnancy and breast feeding. But claims about sluggishly flowing lymph and trapped toxins are unproven.

To the cellulite gurus, a scientific dismissal of their claims will not do. If it is just ordinary fat it can be reduced by conventional means such as diet and exercise, so the cellulitists question the motives of the doctors who deny their claims. In fact most cellulite treatments advocate diet and exercise as part of their programme. Without them any special treatment is unlikely to work.

CHAPTER 5

The Freedom to Eat Well

Whether you're going for an all-out body transformation or just trying to improve your health, your diet is an integral part of your success. Despite what some in the fitness industry may claim, many studies have shown that exercise alone is not very effective in losing weight in a relatively short time unless it is extremely vigorous and frequent. So it's best to combine the two. But the role of diet is frequently misunderstood.

Think Nutrients Over Calories

Food provides the essential ingredients, or nutrients, that your body needs to function properly. Vitamins, minerals and other substances are derived from food to assist virtually everything that goes on in the body. If you don't get the required amount of each of these nutrients, your body will not operate at its best. But even minor deficiencies will affect you in some way: you may feel more tired or bruise more easily than you should. You may look pale or listless and your eyes may be dull instead of sparkling. Your skin may break out in spots, or you may have painful ulcerations in your mouth.

Sure, these are minor problems. But, if you have gone on a diet and deprived yourself of essential nutrient-laden calories to look good, no matter how skinny you get, do you really look or feel good in this state? Picture the anorexic who is supermodel thin. More often than not she looks like a refugee. Hardly anything to aspire to.

I have been a vegetarian for 15 years. During that time my diet hasn't always been healthy, particularly when I was a teenager. I would eat lots of fast food, lots of fried food and lots of cheese to compensate. It was only when I started making a conscious effort to eat many different types of vegetables and fruit, grains and pulses every day that I noticed I looked and felt much better. If I eat a plate of steamed vegetables at night, the next day my complexion will glow. So the first step towards looking and feeling good is to think of nutrients. Then, if you'd like to lose weight you can think of calories.

How Do I Lose Weight By Dieting?

An important distinction between the types of calories you should eat has been made in recent years. It used to be that nutritionists would advise that you cut your intake to lose weight. You could eat whatever you liked as long as it fell within your caloric limit. Now, studies have shown that the different types of calories you eat – fat, protein and carbohydrates – have varying effects on your body.

For example, 100 calories of chocolate cake and 100 calories of banana appear the same but the cake is almost all fat and the banana is nearly all carbohydrate. The 100 calories from the chocolate cake are more likely to be stored as fat somewhere in your body, whereas the carbohydrates from the banana are more likely to be stored in your muscles to be used for quick energy.

If you overeat, excess calories (even if they are from carbohydrates) are likely to be stored as fat. But there is new evidence to suggest

David had been thin as a teenager then suddenly, during university and afterwards, he became quite overweight. He couldn't pinpoint any reason why, except that he wasn't playing football any more although he jogged fairly regularly. It was only when he decided that his drinking was becoming a problem in his life and he stopped, that, to his surprise, over a couple of months, he lost 20 pounds without dieting.

Lesson *Many people drink a few beers or glasses of wine a day. But the accumulated calories can creep up on you. If you drink with dinner three nights a week and have a few drinks at the pub every few days, the extra calories could amount to about 3000 per week. This would cause a weight gain of about 3.5 pounds (1.6 kg) a month or 21 pounds (9.5 kg) over six months! Alcohol may also increase your appetite causing you to eat more as well. Some Swiss researchers found that when people drink alcohol their bodies burn up fat much more slowly than usual.*

high-carbohydrate diet. This would explain why those on a high-carbohydrate diet don't gain weight like those on a high-fat regime of the same number of calories.

The most effective way to lose fat is to lower your fat intake AND decrease your total number of calories. If you are just counting calories, the chances are you're at risk of missing out on vital nutrients. But when you make a conscious effort to eat less fat, you automatically cut out most junk food. What's left is lots of healthy, natural food.

Before you count the calories, think nutrients.

Why Are High-Carbohydrate Diets Best?

There has been much publicity about the importance of a high-carbohydrate diet. When we exercise we use the carbohydrates stored in our muscles. But, because our brain, liver and muscles need carbohydrates to function, the supplies must be restored. Eating a high-carbohydrate diet will ensure that this is done.

In addition, carbohydrates are likely to be used quickly. Even if you don't decrease the amount of calories you eat, a high-carbohydrate diet can aid weight loss. The body increases its metabolic rate to break down the carbohydrates. Finally, even when the carbohydrates are stored as fat, this process uses up almost 25 per cent of the carbohydrate calories consumed. So for every 100 calories of carbohydrates you eat, only 75 may be stored. High-carbohydrate foods are vegetables, fruit, grains, beans and potatoes.

that excess carbohydrates are still better than excess fat. Overeating carbohydrates means they may be burned up, rather than stored as fat. Numerous experts say that your body actually learns to burn calories faster on a

CHAPTER 6

Taking the Hard Work Out of Working Out

Exercise doesn't have to be all grunting, groaning and sweating. These may even be an indication that you're exercising incorrectly. While a few people like to really push themselves, most people prefer exercise to be a gentler experience. Sticking to an exercise plan is both a mental and a physical battle, so finding ways to take the hard work out of working out will increase your ability to deal with the much tougher mental effort.

Choose activities you enjoy instead of forcing yourself to do something that bores you. But giving yourself that extra push *sometimes* is part of the plan. There are some days when I absolutely love to run, and on those occasions it's as if there's no better feeling in the world. Other days, it's all I can do to drag myself on to the treadmill or to the park; but then, once I've started, I end up feeling great. But there are days when I don't even bother and do something else instead. Yet, if every running session was a chore, I'd hardly experience any of the mental benefits which spur me to continue. When exercise makes you feel good, it makes the effort seem that much easier.

Monitoring How You Feel

How hard you push yourself will determine how you feel. This is known as your exercise intensity. Monitoring your exercise intensity can be done in many ways. One way of estimating your oxygen consumption and how hard you are working is to monitor your heart rate. To do this, while exercising take the pulse at your wrist, neck, temple or heart for 6, 10 or 15 seconds and work out the number of beats per minute. The recommended target heart rate is generally between 120 and 170 beats per minute according to your age and fitness level. While this method is a good gauge, it can be difficult to count your pulse correctly, especially during some activities.

Another way is to take the talk test: if you can talk with little difficulty during your workout, then you are probably not working at too high a level.

The easiest method is subjectively determining how you feel at any given moment during exercise using the Borg Scale. In the 1960s Dr Gunnar Borg, a Swedish exercise physiologist, developed a scale of perceived exertion which he found corresponded to various heart rates. Through a numbered scale he designated certain `feelings' to indicate the level of the exerciser's exertion. For example, he began with a number representing effort which felt `very very light'. The numbers at the higher end of his scale reflected exercising at an intensity which felt `heavy' or `very very heavy'.

When developing this test, Borg found that, even though his subjects were all of different fitness levels, if they all felt they were working `somewhat hard', they were all working at the same level of difficulty in relation to their personal fitness level. The numbers corresponded to each individual's appropriate heart rate, or exercise intensity. In other words, they could accurately perceive exactly how hard they were working. Borg's research made clear just how accurate the human barometer is and how much instinctive knowledge we have about our bodies. The current scale being used will be most effective for you if you have already become used to exercise.

How to use the Borg Scale

During your exercise session quickly select a number on the scale that reflects how you feel. Focus on your *overall effort*, not on one sensation such as how tired your calf muscles are. Then you can consciously raise or lower the level of intensity at which you are working. General guidelines recommend that you aim to work at level 4, an intensity which you feel is `somewhat hard'.

Rating	How You Feel
0	Nothing
0.5	Very very light (just noticeable)
1	Very light
2	Light (weak)
3	Moderate
4	Somewhat hard (target heart rate range)
5	Heavy (strong)
6	
7	Very heavy
8	
9	
10	Very very heavy (almost maximum)

Borg's Scale of Perceived Exertion

How Hard Should I Work Out?

The rule is that there *is* no specific rule on how hard you should work out. It depends on what you're trying to achieve. In the past there has been much emphasis on maintaining a certain intensity while you

exercise. Heart monitoring was *de rigueur* in most fitness classes. Since it has now been found that you can experience health benefits from very low levels of intensity, it is not so important to monitor your activity so that you stay within a certain range. The general advice is to work `somewhat hard' during your exercise sessions. If you are trying to burn calories and have a limited amount of time, work at higher intensities. But if working at a higher intensity means you will be sore for days and unlikely to feel motivated to do it again, then you're better off doing something at a low intensity for a little longer. Dramatic fitness training effects usually occur only under higher intensities, but you can still achieve overall health benefits by working out at a low intensity. Be aware of how you feel. If you are new to exercise, keep the intensity low. Allow your body to adapt before you push yourself.

Some people with medical conditions such as heart ailments or hypertension, pregnant women, or those on some medications have an abnormal response to exercise. If you fall into this category, seek medical advice.

Impact vs. Intensity

It is important to realise the difference between impact and intensity. Impact usually refers to the amount of landing force on your joints. *High-impact* activities include those which use pounding or fast movements in which both feet leave the ground temporarily. Jumping, running and high-impact aerobics are high-impact activities. *Low-impact* activities are those where you keep one foot on the ground, or your body weight is supported by something other than your feet during the activity, such as swimming, cycling or using a stair machine.

Intensity refers to how hard you push yourself during a workout. High-impact activities are usually high-intensity too. But low-impact activities can be performed at either high or low intensity. Walking fast or uphill can be high-intensity. If you push your heart to work in the upper ranges of your target heart rate zone, you are said to be working at a high intensity.

Be Soft on Your Body

`No pain, no gain' is a misunderstood and now outdated concept. Pain is usually an indication that the body is being overstressed and perhaps damaged in some way. Although athletes used to be encouraged to work through the pain (i.e. ignore it), we now know better and, if it hurts, we stop. Therein lies the contradiction: there's just no getting around the fact that some exercises *do* hurt.

So how can you tell the difference between good pain and bad pain? There are at least four different kinds of `pain': muscle burning, general fatigue, pain in a localised area, and soreness.

1. Muscle burning

A burning sensation in your muscles is a sign of depleting energy stores and waste accumulating. Because your muscles are contracting over a period of time, your blood flow is stifled. This prevents waste being carried away, allows a build-up of lactic acid and inhibits oxygen from being delivered to the working muscles. With training your muscles will be able to last longer. When you feel a burning sensation in the particular muscle you are working (when doing leg lifts, for example), this is normal muscular fatigue, provided it ceases when you stop the exercise.

If you are doing endurance exercise such as walking, swimming or stepping and you feel burning in your muscles, you should stop or decrease the level of your activity. Since the aim of endurance, or aerobic, activities is to work all the muscles at once

without fatiguing any one group, one group getting tired is a sign you're overdoing it.

If you are doing weight training or calisthenics, which target specific muscles, the muscle burning is an indication that you have reached a point of fatigue. Relax your muscles, then continue with another set if necessary.

2. General fatigue

General fatigue or weakness is a sign that you are tired, dehydrated or depleting your carbohydrate energy stores. While it's not immediately dangerous, you probably need to rest because you are most prone to injuries when fatigued. Eat well and drink water before, during and after your workout.

You may also feel fatigued if you are over-stressed or over-exercising. Allow yourself to relax. Get plenty of sleep.

3. Pain

Pain in a specific area, or even a dull ache, can turn into an acute or chronic injury. When you do an activity such as running or aerobics, where you're not intentionally trying to fatigue a certain muscle group (as in weight lifting), and you feel a specific site of pain such as in a joint, stop exercising immediately. If you are working at the appropriate level of intensity, a specific muscle group should not respond with fatigue.

If you twist your ankle or incur a slight injury while you're exercising, do not ignore it, stop exercising and treat it right away.

4. Soreness

You are bound to feel soreness in your muscles a day or two after strenuous exercise, resistance exercises or when performing a new type of movement. If you are so sore you have difficulty doing *anything* the next day, you've been working too hard. Decrease the intensity of your next few workouts. If your legs get sore and tired, switch to an upper body workout for a few days, or vice versa. If you are *continually* sore, you probably are not allowing enough recovery time in between workouts.

> Jenny had a niggling pain in her leg, also known as `shin splints'. It usually hurt in the morning but by the time she was into her run or aerobics class it felt OK. Over a few months' time it worsened and it soon became painful during her workouts. She decided to give it a rest and stopped exercising for two weeks. When she resumed it felt a little better but a few weeks later it got so bad she went to the doctor. It turned out she had developed a stress fracture and had to stop exercising for eight weeks.
>
> **Lesson** *Many committed exercisers find it impossible to slow down or rest when they have niggles of pain. They rationalise the pain and think that somehow they can work it off. The fact is, if your body is sore it's a sign that there is some degree of injury which needs healing. Decrease the intensity and frequency of what you're doing now so you won't have to give up entirely later. Any sort of repetitive exercise is prone to injury so it's best to keep variety in your workout.*

Better Safe than Sorry

Exercise safety has been the single most publicised issue in the fitness industry. Although exercise today is safer than it has ever been, widespread media coverage exaggerating the dangerous elements has given some activities, such as running, aerobics and step, a very bad name. In fact, technological advances have shown the effects of different movements on the body and have led to a much better understanding of injuries and the most effective ways to train.

The rule of thumb is that if an exercise puts potentially harmful stress on a body part, the risks outweigh the benefit of the move. The exercises included in this list are some of the most common exercises that have been practised for centuries in sports and dance training. However, deep knee bends, double leg lifts while lying on your back, full sit-ups, bouncing stretches, the yoga plough, the hurdler stretch and excessive unsupported bending of the spine in any direction are all considered risky. While a professional athlete or dancer may have to do some of these moves, experts recommend that most exercisers avoid them.

Why do I sometimes have trouble breathing?

When you inhale, oxygen is carried to the tiny air sacs in your lungs. It takes a fraction of a second for the passing blood in the capillaries to grab on to the oxygen molecules to transport them where needed in the body. If you are working too hard, your breathing rate speeds up making it more difficult for this transfer to occur, so you may get less oxygen where it's needed.

Breathe as naturally and as slowly as possible during any aerobic exercise. Try to avoid breathing loudly in time with the music in an aerobics class, instead breathe slower than the beat of the music. When lifting weights it is important, though, to control your breathing to prevent a rise in internal pressure. Exhale on the muscular effort and inhale on the release.

As you become fitter the number of blood cells in your body increases. This and other physiological adaptations means you can work harder and faster. But no matter how fit you are, if you start gasping it's a sign you're working above your level.

But not everyone adheres to these guidelines. Many people feel that if it doesn't hurt when you do it, it's OK. In fact, these movements won't usually cause immediate injuries. They just contribute to long-term wear and tear of the body. Just because you *can* do them, doesn't mean you *should*.

While people exercise for many reasons, the main aim of *true fitness* is to improve physical well-being. You may play a sport for variety, dance for fun and do high-intensity work on the aerobics machines to burn calories, but the underlying assumption must be that it is all done with safety as the first consideration. Bearing that in mind, any actions which may jeopardise your body should be eliminated.

Although more and more fitness and aerobics classes are heeding the rules, outside the professional exercise studio there are dance classes, yoga workouts, fitness videos and sports which incorporate some, if not all, of these potentially dangerous exercises. This is because these disciplines develop what is known as functional fitness. While they can help you achieve good health, their primary motive is to develop the skills and fitness needed to practise that activity. In striving for these very different goals, potentially harmful moves may be used as part of the training or repertoire of moves in the activity.

If you predominantly use one side of your body to kick a ball or execute a tennis serve, even though you may be developing an imbalanced musculature which may hurt your spine, these actions are required for these particular sports. In gymnastics, the hyperflexibility required can be extremely detrimental to all the joints, but is necessary to perform all gymnastics moves. In dance, the body is put in many stressful positions in order to express concepts or the emotions in the music. Those who practise any of these activities assume the risks inherent in the sport. You'd be hard pressed to find any professional athlete or dancer *without* a chronic injury or weakness. If you are in a group that performs these moves, don't be embarrassed to refrain from doing something you know to be stressful.

So how are you to know what to do and what not to do? In Chapter 14 I've listed a few of the most common risky exercises which should be avoided. However, any exercise or activity can be unsafe if performed incorrectly, without a sufficient warm-up, or in unstable conditions.

Your best bet is to seek advice and check up on it periodically to watch for any new developments. For example, step and sliding are such new activities that results of research are still emerging. Some of the techniques being used today might next year be considered too stressful. So find out from qualified sources: certified fitness instructors and books and videos presented by fitness educators (not celebrities) with an academic background in the field and current teaching certifications. Chapter 11 lists the internationally recognised fitness instructor certifications your teacher should have.

Outside Factors

Weather conditions can challenge your workouts. If it's hot, you need to acclimatise yourself slowly to the heat and drink plenty of water. Some people worry that if you drink water while exercising it will cause cramps or nausea. In fact, you can get dehydrated and sick from *not* drinking water, especially when it is very hot or humid. You should take sips of water at regular intervals before, during and after the exercise period.

In cold weather you want to preserve your body heat. Keep your head, hands and feet covered. Since your body may take longer to warm up, move into the activity more slowly than usual.

CHAPTER 7

Strategy Curves

Curves is based on the principle that a fitness programme must curve, or fluctuate, to respond to your changing needs along the way. If it doesn't, you will not achieve your potential.

Now that you have an idea of how the body works, here are a few exercise fundamentals to apply to your programme as and when you need them. These basic fitness training principles, or Strategy Curves, demonstrate how you should adapt your fitness programme to new situations which will arise in your fitness routine. The 12-week Body Transformation Curves will adapt to your individual needs if you allow the following Strategy Curves to dictate your progress.

The Gentle Curve

Start at your own level and progress accordingly.

More is not always better. There is a law of diminishing returns in exercise. If you do too much, at the very least you are a candidate for burn-out and at worst, you will be injured. Exercise puts stress on all parts of your body. By working harder you'll become stronger. It's a gradual process, though: too much stress too soon results in body fatigue or injury.

Moderate amounts of exercise improve your ability to fight illness by boosting your immune cells. But exercising at strenuous levels increases your production of cortisol and adrenaline – stress hormones which suppress your immune system. So too much may mean you also get ill more often.

Exercise at your own pace. This means if you are taking an aerobics class for the first time, find a beginners' class that suits your level of fitness and skill. Even if you are already fit from another activity, you still need to start at an introductory level when you do something new.

It's very easy to do too much if you work out with a partner. In trying to keep up you may be compelled to work at a much harder level than you should. This often happens with couples who run together, even if they are both at the same fitness level. The taller person will have a naturally longer stride, so the shorter person will have to exert much more effort just to keep the same pace.

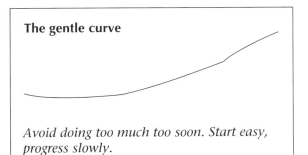

The gentle curve

Avoid doing too much too soon. Start easy, progress slowly.

The Bull's-Eye Curve

As explained in Chapter 2, to get specific results you need to follow a training programme specifically designed to achieve them. You cannot follow one path to several different goals, you must choose the necessary route to each.

This is true when you want to improve any

one of the main components of fitness: flexibility, muscular strength, muscular endurance, cardiovascular endurance, and body composition (muscle to fat ratio). But it also applies to specific co-ordination and athletic skills. If you want to improve your tennis serve, jogging won't help much. But practising the serve over and over again and strengthening the muscles involved in serving will.

Not being specific is where I have seen most people go wrong. Because of the lack of widely available information about the results a certain programme can achieve, I have seen women attending stretch classes five days a week or practising Callanetics in the hope of losing weight. Or I have seen men do countless repetitions of sit-ups to trim their waistlines. While it's an achievement to do *any* exercise, and you are sure to experience some benefits whatever you do, you are apt to get highly discouraged if you don't reach your specific goal. So start targeting.

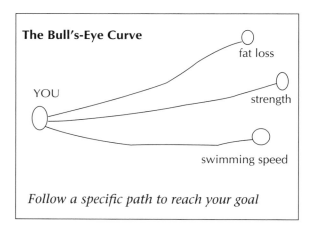

The Bull's-Eye Curve

fat loss

YOU

strength

swimming speed

Follow a specific path to reach your goal

The Body Learning Curve

The more you exercise, the more you will learn about how your body responds to an activity. It's crucial that you listen to your body and adapt your programme according to the signals it gives you. Am I out of breath? Is the activity so light I'm not even breaking a sweat? Is there a niggling pain in my knee? Was that a good, solid squash hit

from my whole body or one that hit the wrong part of the racket where power was propelled more from my wrist?

There is a tendency to focus outwards during any activity – especially during those where you are purposely distracted such as sports, aerobics and dance classes. This can prove detrimental if your body sends you a signal you don't hear. In an aerobics class you can get so caught up trying to figure out the steps, you may not be totally aware of the sensations each step creates in your body. At the very least, you miss out on some of the pleasurable sensations, but you may also be more susceptible to injury.

It's very easy to focus on your body and then misinterpret what you feel. A common mistake is to do double leg lifts to work the abdomen: this is an exercise where you lie flat on your back, then lift and lower both straight legs about six inches off the ground. This exercise has the reputation of being very advanced – a tough abdominal workout. When you do it you do indeed feel the strain, but the strain is not in your abdominal muscles, it's in your lower back and hip muscles in the front of your upper thighs. Most people fail to recognise this.

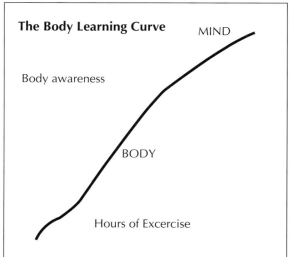

The Body Learning Curve　　MIND

Body awareness

BODY

Hours of Excercise

The more you exercise, the more you'll learn about your body. Monitor your workouts accordingly.

The Overload Curve

As you exercise, your body becomes stronger. It also enables you to do increasing levels of exercise: you can do an aerobics class without getting as tired as you did when you first started; you can walk further; you can lift more weights. In order to keep improving, the body must be subjected to controlled overload. That is, there must be a progressive increased stress on the muscles and system involved. If not, the body will respond by maintaining, but not improving, its current fitness level. Have you ever hit a plateau while following a programme? You may have experienced results at first but after a while nothing more seemed to happen. It could have been that your body successfully adapted to the challenge you gave it at first but when you ceased to keep challenging it, it ceased to keep adapting.

You can increase the overload by manipulating the frequency, intensity or duration of your exercise. This may mean that during your programme, if you feel you are able to complete each of your sessions very easily, you may want to add another day per week. Or you could push yourself harder – walk faster, or concentrate on resisting with your arms more during aerobics, for example. It's best to vary the ways in which you stress your body. For instance, you may decide to overload by increasing the duration of your workout or activity by five minutes each week. If you start walking for 30 minutes, several months later you could be walking up to two hours a session. Obviously this is impractical for most people and might cause you to drop out rather than continue. A better approach would be to walk a little longer on some days, a little faster on other days, travel over more hills on some days, and cycle on others.

There's a limit on your overload. If you try to increase at a drastic rate in order to get quick results, it can backfire. There are certain bodily processes you cannot speed up. Muscle conditioning, for example, requires that you allow 48-hours rest in between resistance training sessions so your muscles have time to heal and become stronger. In some cases an elite athlete may recover more quickly than this and therefore be able to work the muscles more often. But most people need the full recovery time. If you push it and work the same muscle groups very intensely every day rather than giving them a break, you may hurt yourself, or at least hamper the rate of your improvement.

Fat loss, too, cannot be speeded up. You have hundreds of thousands of fat calories stored in your body. Every time you exercise for 30 minutes you may use 200-400 calories (depending on what you do). You can see that 200 out of hundreds of thousands of calories is barely going to make a dent in your fat stores. Not until you have used several thousands of calories over a period of months will you see a noticeable difference in body shape from the *outside*. You simply cannot hurry the process, because it is virtually impossible to use up the calories any quicker. Obviously dieting will help build up a caloric dent, but there's even a limit on that. For the body is adept at the art of survival and, if you starve yourself, it will hold on to the fat in various ways, including slowing down your metabolism.

As you can see from the gentle upward-sloping overload curve, the key here is to overload *gradually* so your body has time to adapt to the changing stimuli before you increase the stress still further. As you get older, your body takes longer to adapt so you may want to go even more slowly than you used to.

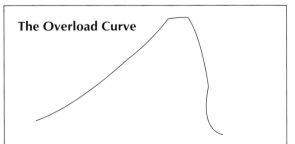

The Overload Curve

To improve, there must be progressive, but gradual, increased stress on your body

Janet has been walking an hour a day to and from work for over a year. She does high-impact aerobic classes (two to four times a month). She occasionally practises to an exercise video and had one month where she swam once a week. She wants to strengthen her legs (particularly her inner thighs) and abdomen and to lose fat, but she feels that nothing seems to work.

Lesson *Janet's case is simple. Although she is right to keep a variety in her workouts, and her walks are helping her overall health, she is not consistent. In order to effect a change on her body shape she needs to do more and stick to it.*

The Cross Training Curve

Cross training is a form of programming where, instead of sticking to one activity, you `cross over' and include several others in your schedule. The most well-known form of cross training is the triathlon where you run, bike and swim in one race. The way you cross train can vary immensely. You can simply do several different activities each week (as scheduled in the Body Transformation Curves). Or you can perform specific activities which hone in on different components of fitness (flexibility, muscular strength, co-ordination) or rotate different high- and low-impact sports. Or if you are an athlete training for a certain sport, you may plan a more complex schedule where, in addition to your main sport, you phase in a different activity for a number of weeks, then add a new one.

The idea behind cross training is that by switching over to various activities, you also vary the stresses on your body. This often means less injury risk since most sports injuries are due to overuse and the strain of a repetitive movement. You also can gain better all-round fitness because you are not just developing a specific ability in one activity, but in a number of them. Often these will be complementary and strengthen different areas of your body: rowing may develop your upper body while cycling favours the lower body; weight training can give you the all-round balanced muscular strength that running alone simply cannot. An athlete may also find cross training useful because he or she can rest from the stress of their regular training without sacrificing their overall fitness level.

You may also burn more calories. Since your body responds to exercise by getting more efficient at producing energy for an activity, you ultimately work less hard and burn fewer calories once your body has adapted (this is why you need to overload). When you cross train, because your body is always adapting to new forms of stress, it may never become fully efficient at any one.

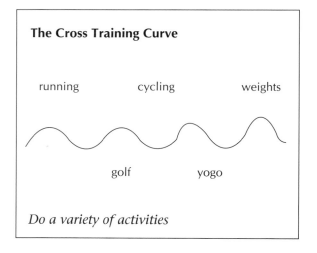

The Cross Training Curve

running   cycling   weights

golf   yogo

Do a variety of activities

Keep these exercise principles in mind to remember that exercise is not a rigid plan but a programme which will be individual to you. You are now ready to learn more about the *Curves* Strategy and design the right Curve for you.

Pat had been slightly overweight for many years. For the past five years she had dabbled in a variety of diets and exercise programmes. She had also been power walking for 45 minutes, three days a week all those years. Her body weight stayed the same. She finally concluded that she had tried everything and that liposuction was the only answer. She had it done and was severely bruised for months afterwards. She couldn't exercise during this period at all. A year later she had gained even more weight.

Lesson *Pat was on the brink of mental burn-out. Although she was quite disciplined in sticking to a programme for five years, she saw no measurable changes in her body shape. Her mistake was simple: she did not keep adapting her programme to her changing body and also did not undertake enough high calorie-burning and fat-loss activity. She learned the hard way that liposuction is not the answer. For, even if fat cells are removed, there is no guarantee that new ones will not grow back. Even if they don't, unless you're eating and exercising regularly, the fat will just be stored elsewhere in the body.*

PART TWO

THE FOUR 'Ps'

Now that you understand how to achieve your goal, Part Two will show you how, by taking the Four Ps into account, to choose the right activities for you - your personality, psychology, physical needs and practical considerations.

CHAPTER 8

The Body Transformation Strategy

Curves is based on a method I devised to design fitness programmes for my personal clients. It's a step-by-step formula which takes goals, needs, likes and limitations into account. When you exercise, you cannot simply decide to follow a static plan. Curving, rather than remaining rigid, is the key to your success. First, the programme must be suited to you and meet your individual needs. The next three chapters will look at the four Ps: aspects of your personality; the psychology behind what motivates you; physical considerations – you need to take into account to ensure the exercise is safe for your body; and practical matters that will influence how well you exercise.

There are a variety of programmes you can follow. You must first determine which one leads to your goal, then personalise it according to your individual needs. To transform your body, the programme must be progressive in order to achieve results. What you do in the first week will gradually increase in intensity over the weeks as your body adapts to the new exercise and becomes more fit. The Body Learning Curve (Chapter 7) will help you modify it as needed along the way. Each programme lasts for 12 weeks, by which time you will have begun to see real results. You will have progressed to a higher level of movement and fitness and will look and feel much better. If you aim to improve your health or energy levels or reduce stress, then you should achieve this goal by the end of 12 weeks. If you are trying to lose weight and reshape your body, you will certainly have started to tone up and

lose fat. How much fat you lost depends upon the intensity of the programme you followed. You may need to continue with another 12 weeks of the programme to see more results. This is explained further in Chapter 17.

The Body Transformation Strategy

1. Identify your individual traits. Based on the four Ps – personality, psychological, physical and practical – choose the activities most suited to you.

2. Choose the activities you'd most like to do.

3. Divide your chosen activities into intensity and impact levels. Keep in mind any medical advice you have been given.

4. Pick the Body Transformation Curve you would most like to follow (Health, Energy, Body or Serenity). Read the appropriate chapter and, using the blank schedules provided, substitute the activities from your list where appropriate.

5. Start moving!

Identify your individual traits. Based on the four Ps – personality, psychological, physical and practical – choose the activities most suited to you.

Look at the following characteristics. Decide which best describes you most of the time and include the designated activities on your list. You may find that seemingly opposing characteristics apply to you at different times or moods in your life. Try to pick the predominant one. If you feel it is too hard to pick just one then go ahead and choose both sets of activities.

List all activities associated with a certain trait. Even if you have never participated in one before or do not enjoy it, you can weed it out later.

The activities listed are those which are most accessible to most people: a detailed description of each activity is given in Appendix A.

Personality Traits

1. Are you mostly a social extrovert or are you more introverted and enjoy solitary activities?

Social	Solitary	List
running clubs	running	_____
walking groups	walking/hiking	_____
cycling clubs	cycling	_____
tennis	*fitness classes	_____
squash	swimming	_____
basketball	video workouts	_____
soccer		_____
golf		_____
badminton		_____
most sports		_____

* Attending fitness classes can be social or solitary. In most cases, however, it is solitary as there is little group interaction.

2. Weather permitting, would you prefer an outdoor activity, even though it may be less convenient? Or would you be more likely to use the nearest leisure facilities?

Personality Traits

Outdoors	Indoors	List
running/walking outdoors	running/walking on a treadmill	_____
tennis outdoors	tennis indoors	_____
football	squash	_____
rugby	fitness classes	_____
swimming outdoors	swimming indoors	_____
cycling outdoors	stationary cycle	_____
ice skating	aqua aerobics	_____
golf	dance classes	_____
rollerblading	other fitness equipment	_____
other outdoor sports	video workouts	_____

3. Variety is good for some, monotony good for others. Do you get bored easily? Or do you play the same tape over and over again, like to eat the same foods?

Variety	Repetition	List
step classes	stair machine	_____
running outside/races	treadmill walking	_____
cycling tours	cycling indoors	_____
mountain climbing	Versiclimber	_____
cross-country skiing	Nordik trak	_____
basketball	swimming	_____
soccer	treadmill running	_____
squash		_____
tennis		_____
rollerblading		_____
golf		_____
dance classes		_____
fitness classes		_____
other sports		_____

Personality Traits

4. Are you very analytical? Do you like activities that you can do without having to develop a lot of skills beforehand? Or do you like to learn something thoroughly?

Simple	Complex	List
conditioning exercises	martial arts	_____
weight training	golf	_____
walking/running	fitness classes	_____
swimming	tennis/squash	_____
cycling	soccer	_____
yoga	dance classes	_____
aerobic machines	sports	_____

5. Do you like competitive activities that charge you up? Or do you get highly emotional and feel the need to work off aggression? Do you need to relax and relieve stress?

Competitive	Emotional Release	List
tennis	dance classes	_____
running races	running alone	_____
squash	fitness classes	_____
basketball	weight training	_____
soccer	swimming	_____
most sports		_____

6. Are you playful or very serious?

Playful	Serious	List
all sports	solitary activities (walking,	_____
group events (cycle ride,	running, cycling)	_____
walking clubs)	martial arts	_____
rollerblading	yoga	_____
ice skating		_____
aqua aerobics		_____
rebounding, mini		_____
trampoline		_____

Personality Traits

7. Do you see physical activity as an enjoyable diversion from other areas of your life? Or do you see it as your private time and get inspired?

Pleasurable Escape	Meditative	List
group activities	walking/running	_____
sports	yoga	_____
fitness classes	martial arts	_____
golf	stretching	_____
video workouts	Pilates	_____
dance classes	aerobic machines	_____

8. Do you prefer to be guided through exercise so you don't have to decide what to do? Or do you prefer to be in control of it?

External motivator/instruction	Self disciplined	List
fitness classes (modern and jazz dance, ballet)	solitary activities (running, cycling, walking, swimming, rowing)	_____
aqua aerobics		_____
weight training	weight training	_____
yoga	video workouts	_____
Pilates	aerobic machines	_____
personal trainer		

9. Now go through and consolidate your list.

LIST A

_____	_____	_____	_____	_____
_____	_____	_____	_____	_____
_____	_____	_____	_____	_____
_____	_____	_____	_____	_____
_____	_____	_____	_____	_____
_____	_____	_____	_____	_____
_____	_____	_____	_____	_____
_____	_____	_____	_____	_____
_____	_____	_____	_____	_____

Now turn to the next chapter so you can start to personalise your list further.

CHAPTER 9

What Makes You Tick?

PSYCHOLOGICAL

Obviously, not all of the personality traits listed in Chapter 8 are equal. Being social may be more important to you than having an outside person motivate you. Or your competitive streak may be stronger than your desire to be meditative and reflect while you work out. Keeping this in mind, go through the following considerations to specialise your list.

1. Do you see new activities as exciting and worth the risk? Or do you get slightly frightened at the prospect of trying an unknown sport and prefer to stick to things you are already comfortable with? Go through your list and cross off those activities you know you would definitely not attempt.

2. What are your mental barriers? In the preceding list you may have come across areas where you realised a weakness. Are you too serious? Too introverted? Perhaps these are character traits you would like to overcome. Go back through the list and add activities that you think might develop your desired qualities.

3. Do you have an addictive or compulsive personality? Are there some activities which you know would exacerbate rather than help this tendency? Cross these activities from your list.

4. Do you get overly emotional and have problems dealing with anger? Would some competitive sports make you more upset than happy? Cross these activities from your list.

5. Have you had a negative experience with exercise in the past? Were you made fun of in sports and games at school? If so, you may wish to do non–sport activities and build your fitness up in other ways (walking, gym, exercise machines, cycling). When you have developed physical strength and self–confidence you could consider tackling some of the activities you felt uncomfortable with in the past.

6. Have you ever exercised and been so sore for days afterwards that you wouldn't try the activity again? If so, reconsider what you now know about exercise training. Did you overload too much? Was there a mistake you made that you could avoid if you tried the activity again?

7. What weight loss methods have you tried before? How did your body respond? What caused the regain? Do you see any activities that may help now?

8. Are you achievement–oriented – do you like to have proof of what you have accomplished? Go through your list and identify how you can make your potential activities achievement–oriented. (Running races as opposed to running on a treadmill, playing sports rather than just taking an aerobics class.) On the other hand, if you are not very competitive, your marks of achievement could be something other than winning. They could simply be

accomplishing an activity every day for a week, or going a certain distance.

9. List your likes and dislikes. Cross off anything on your list that you absolutely detest. If you're unsure, leave it on.

10. Which personal habits may inhibit your progress (smoking, prescription drugs, late nights for instance)? How can you change them or work around them?

Adjust your list for any other psychological considerations you noticed during this exercise.

LIST B

CHAPTER 10

Your Special Needs

PHYSICAL CONSIDERATIONS

Since you want the exercise you do to help, rather than hurt, you, it's vital to take your physical needs into account. Answer the following questions to help identify any physical considerations which may be affected by working out. Exclude the activities which may exacerbate them. Include the activities which may help them.

Some conditions require that you eliminate certain activities. Other conditions require that you modify the way you perform an activity. For example, if you have a heart problem you can still walk but you must adjust the intensity at which you work. If you have a back condition you may do aerobics, but might prefer low impact as opposed to high impact. Or if you choose to run, you might do so on grass rather than pavement. If you are pregnant, the exercise intensity you should follow depends upon your pre-pregnancy fitness level.

It is always advisable to consult your doctor before beginning any new exercise programme. If you have an existing medical condition, you should contact the appropriate specialist for advice and precautions.

These are just a few of the physical problems to be aware of. Once you find out how to arrange your programme around them, continue on the Body Transformation Strategy. Eliminate any activities you most certainly cannot do from List B in Chapter 9.

Please check with your doctor if you have suffered from any of the following conditions or are taking prescribed medication. Your doctor may not ask you to refrain from exercising, since in many cases (arthritis, some heart trouble, asthma for instance) exercise can help your condition. But you may have to make certain modifications to your programme.

Aids
anaemia
angina
arthritis
asthma
blood pressure problems
cancer
chronic bronchitis
chronic cough, coughing up blood
constipation, diarrhoea, ulcers
cramps in your body
diabetes
difficulty breathing
emphysema
epilepsy
heart trouble
insomnia, excessive fatigue
lung cancer
menopause symptoms
migraines or recurrent headaches
multiple sclerosis
nervous/emotional problems
numbness in your hands or feet
obesity
pains, tightness, discomfort or palpitations of heart and chest
pneumonia
pre-existing back condition
pre-existing knee or other joint problems
pre-existing muscular problems
pregnancy
respiratory problems
rheumatic fever
stroke or cardiovascular disease
swollen ankles
thyroid problems
tuberculosis
varicose veins
vision/hearing problems

Choose what you'd most like to do

With your revised list assess your possible activity choices. Differentiate between those you would be most and least likely to do.

Read Chapter 11 and Appendix A for more information about your possible activity choices. Put a star beside those activities you would be likely to do immediately. Put a tick next to those which you might be willing to try or do occasionally. If an activity simply does not appeal to you at all, cross it off.

Divide your chosen activities into intensity and impact levels. Keep in mind any medical advice you have been given.

Make sure none of the activities you have chosen is potentially harmful to you. You may wish to eliminate exercises which are of too high an intensity or impact for your specific condition. Some activities can be performed at different intensities depending on how hard you work. Go back and review Chapter 7 on monitoring your exercise intensity.

The Chart below divides various activities into a general intensity and impact level. This is just a guideline; your own fitness level and performance will determine the true intensity of your workouts.

Go through your final list and mark next to each activity whether it is:

> Low Intensity, High Impact (LIHI)
> High Intensity, High Impact (HIHI)
> Low Intensity, Low Impact (LILI)
> High Intensity, Low Impact (HILI)

This will be useful if you want to substitute

Intensity and Impact Levels of Different Types of Exercise

Low Intensity, High Impact (LIHI)	Low Intensity, Low Impact (LILI)	High Intensity, Low Impact (HILI)	Conditioning (Con)
tennis	aqua aerobics	badminton	calisthenics/stretch
walking/jogging	ballroom dancing	cycling indoors	and tone classes
	cardiofunk	hiking	Pilates
	cardiosculpting	ice skating	weight training
High Intensity, High Impact (HIHI)	cycling outdoors	modern dancing	yoga
	golf	Nordik trak	
American football	LI aerobics	pool running	
basketball	modern and jazz	rollerblading	
circuit class	dance, ballet	slide	
high-impact	rebounding	stair machine	
aerobics	rowing	step	
running	swimming	treadmill walking	
skipping with a rope	tai chi	on an incline	
soccer	walking	Versiclimber	
squash	weight training		

an activity on the fitness plan with one you have chosen as especially suitable to your personality, psychological, physical and practical needs.

PRACTICAL CONSIDERATIONS

Obviously there are many practical considerations which will determine what you can do: you may love running races but there may not be as many opportunities as you'd like. Or there may not be a yoga class that is convenient for you. Apply each of the following questions to each activity on your list. Adjust your list as necessary.

1. Can I afford this activity?
2. Must I learn a skill before I can practice this activity? Is instruction available nearby?
3. Is it convenient? If I am tired and have worked late, will it be too far or too much of a hassle to motivate myself to do on a regular basis? What facilities can I use? Do I live near a park?
4. Are there factors which may inhibit my doing this activity? (Pollution or traffic for outdoor pursuits? No one to watch the children?) Can I compensate in some way? (Do it only at weekends, in the mornings? Hire a babysitter?)
5. What equipment do I have already? (Home exercise equipment, fitness videos, a bicycle?)
6. What equipment do I need to buy? (Proper trainers, clothing, etc?)
7. Realistically speaking, how often will I exercise? Rather than make grandiose plans I know I can't keep, how can I schedule my exercise sessions so that I make sure I do them? (Keep potential disruptions in mind so that you can avoid them and stick to your plan.)

Now devise your final list of activities to include in your Curve exercise plan. These activities are ones you will be most likely to

FINAL LIST

enjoy and/or stick to because you have done them before or they are accessible in some way. When you begin the appropriate Curve Strategy, you may substitute these for some

If you want to:	Follow this:
• Improve your overall health; decrease your risk of long-term diseases	Health Curve
• Improve your endurance/stamina; increase your energy levels and ability to do everyday activities	Energy Curve
• Lose weight or body fat; resculpt your body, improve strength and muscle tone	Body Curve
• Reduce stress; improve your mental well-being	Serenity Curve

of the activities on the plan. You may also add some new ones you'd like to try.

Pick the Body Transformation Curve you would most like to follow. Read the appropriate chapter, and using the blank schedules provided, substitute the activities from your list where appropriate.

THE HEALTH CURVE

For many years most people believed that you had to do some sort of fairly strenuous aerobic exercise at least three times a week for at least 30 continuous minutes to reap any benefits. Recent studies have now revised this thinking. Some have shown that improvements in health can be obtained with relatively little activity, even a 20-30 minute session of low-intensity activity such as gardening or walking just a few days a week. And it doesn't have to be taken at once. You can walk to the shops for 10 minutes, do some gardening for 15 minutes and go up and down a few flights of stairs, or vacuum, for five minutes. Adding *any* activity to your life can improve your health.

It's never too late to start. A study in the *New England Journal of Medicine* found that middle-aged and elderly men (45-84 years) who take up moderately vigorous activities such as tennis, swimming, jogging or brisk walking have a 23-29 per cent lower overall death rate and up to a 41 per cent reduction in the risk of coronary artery disease than non-exercisers. In addition, many studies have shown that moderate exercise can actually boost your immune system, thereby making you less susceptible to both serious and everyday illnesses. In short, doing anything is better than doing nothing.

If you want to reshape your body or lose weight, then you'll need to do a bit more exercise than is given on this Curve. To simply improve your health, this programme will focus on frequent bouts of low-intensity exercise. Remember you can substitute some of the activities in this 12 week programme with those from your list but the key is to intersperse as much easy activity into your normal lifestyle as possible.

THE ENERGY CURVE

My father always tells me he's too tired to exercise. He claims that since he doesn't have enough energy, he needs to conserve it so he can do his normal day-to-day activities. I haven't managed to convince him that, although you may feel tired when you start exercising, it's almost guaranteed that you will feel energised by the end of your session. There are both immediate and long-term energy-giving benefits. The immediate effects are simply the result of blood pumping faster through your body and the subsequent release of stress hormones surging into your bloodstream. The more intense your exercise, the more of a high you will feel.

The long-term training effects of an aerobic-based programme are due to the increased efficiency of your body. Put simply, if your body works better, you are going to feel better. The worse shape you are in physically, the more apt you are not to notice. Compare it to driving an old junky car and a brand new Mercedes: in the old car lots of things rattle, hum and clank about and you might not notice the poor shock absorption or uncomfortable seats because you are used to them; a finely tuned Mercedes, on the other hand, is so smooth and efficient that the minute something goes wrong you feel it or hear it right away.

The Energy Curve is designed to get your major systems back in smooth running order. It includes an aerobic element so that you can increase your stamina, improve the efficiency of your heart, lower your blood pressure and reap other internal benefits. There is also an anaerobic element so that you can be prepared for extra stress or calls for energy which you may need sporadically during the day. Finally, there is a muscle-conditioning component so that you can increase your muscular endurance and strength. For instance, if you are moving furniture, you're more likely to be able to do it comfortably. Or, if you are walking home from the shops carrying heavy bags, you will be able to do it easily. Rest is also a very important, and often forgotten, component. If you don't have enough sleep you won't have enough energy, since it is during sleep and meditative states that our body heals and revitalises.

Beware of the energy depleters:

- **Too little sleep** Sleep is an undervalued nutrient. Not getting enough can impair both your mental and athletic performance. You'll feel fatigued, irritable and have a hard time concentrating.

- **Smoking** decreases your oxygen supply to body tissues.

- **Stress** drains mental and physical energy.

- **Too much exercise** uses up your carbohydrate stores.

- **Dehydration** Lack of water can make you tired. If you drink primarily teas, colas and alcohol you may be dehydrating yourself without knowing it.

- **Not enough food** Your food gives you energy. An especially low carbohydrate intake can make you very tired

- **Big meals, infrequent meals** Eating large quantities can send you into a siesta stupor; going hungry causes drops in blood sugar which make you feel tired

THE BODY CURVE

If your intention is to lose fat and reshape your body, this is the Curve to follow. As explained earlier in the book, the key is to burn enough calories and develop enough muscle mass so that you use up fat stores while developing a firm body.

Compared to all the other Curves, this one requires the most commitment and must be combined with a low-fat eating plan. There is no need to starve, just watch your overall calorie intake. It may take a while to see the results you want so this is not a `get-thin-quick' scheme. If you are consistent you can definitely transform your body. How long it takes depends entirely on what condition you are in when you start. If you are fairly fit already and not overweight, then you may wish to concentrate on more muscle-conditioning work. If you are overweight, then your emphasis should primarily be on using up calories, so you may need to do more aerobic work than conditioning.

The exercise should be undertaken at as high an intensity as you can work out safely. The lower the intensity, the longer you'll need to work out in order to effect the maximum calorie loss. Where you lose the fat from is going to depend on where your fat stores are and how far you are into the programme. Generally, upper-body fat is lost first, and abdominal fat is usually much easier to decrease than lower-body fat stores. When doing resistance training, you will first notice increases in muscular strength, but your muscles will not start to increase in size until after about three months of consistent training.

The Body Curve incudes a variety of calorie-burning endurance activities as well as intensive muscle-conditioning exercises with resistance.

THE SERENITY CURVE

If you wish to reduce stress and improve your mental well-being you should follow this Curve. It's only recently that the relationship between mind and body has been acknowledged. It's a growing field of study with even the medical world now researching the mind's effect on the body. Exercise has many important immediate and long-term psychological effects. It improves your mood, decreases mild anxiety, stress and depression while enhancing self-esteem and self-confidence. Cycling or running for at least 60 minutes releases mood-enhancing brain endorphins. Yoga induces a peaceful, anxiety-reducing calm. Aerobic exercise has helped to improve the condition of people suffering from depression. In a recent study, American cardiologist Dr James Rippe found that, after a group of men and women had followed a six-week course of brisk walking, their mood had changed for the better, and anxiety, stress and depression were reduced. Many studies have found that exercise and a positive mood are directly related, irrespective of the degree of cardiovascular fitness.

If you have a highly stressful work situation, troubled family life, or are prone to getting emotional, angry or depressed too often, exercise won't change the situation. What it will do is help you cope.

The Serenity Curve includes some aerobic work which will help your mind deal with stress. It also includes some 'thinking exercise' such as yoga or meditative techniques which will help you learn to distance yourself from your problems so that they can be seen in a healthier, larger perspective.

If you have a specific goal

There are several goals for which you will need to devise training regimens which are much more specific than the Body Transformation Curves in this book. If you want to improve certain sports abilities or develop specific skills such as martial arts or dance, you'll need to consult the appropriate teachers. It will be beneficial to follow one of the basic Curves to help you develop your strength and fitness. Then you will have a solid base for doing more specific work related to your activity. Consult the relevant expert in order to find a step-by-step plan. See Appendix B for useful addresses.

Start moving!

Perform the warm-up stretches in Chapter 16 and begin your chosen programme. Don't forget to read the last four chapters to find out how to stay motivated.

CHAPTER 11

Choices

Inside or Out? Sport or Fitness?

Picture the ancient Greek athlete entering today's hi-tech health club. The Olympic founding fathers could never have imagined what fitness training would become. No more heaving rocks and hurdling grassy knolls: today, urban athletes enter sunless compounds and flex their bodies to the tune of synchronised music and computerised equipment. There are even virtual reality exercise video games. But traditionalists believe that, for the average participant, the old way is better.

The old way means outdoor activities. Whether you play a competitive sport or gallivant through a forest on foot or by bike, the focus is on enjoying the activity. Well-developed muscles are more practical than pretty.

As well as being free of charge and convenient (depending upon the sport), training outdoors is usually more interesting. No matter how sophisticated the computer graphics are, or how loud the MTV, there is an inescapable tedium to machines that go nowhere. After all, they're work. Outdoor play provides just enough stimuli for your mind to forget the physical stress. In an ideal world you can get just as fit outdoors.

Experts agree that total fitness means good muscle strength and endurance, flexibility, aerobic stamina, co-ordination, power and speed. You can develop all these components of physical fitness in some outdoor activities and sports, but there are usually some imbalances. If all you did was to run, for example, you might lack upper-body strength or overall co-ordination. There are well-balanced disciplines – martial arts, dance and gymnastics – but since some of the moves they do are stressful, there's an element of risk in the long term. Also the competitive

Myth

Swimming is the best exercise

False. Many people advocate certain forms of exercise over others. It may be that someone is trying to promote their own product or technique, so be discerning when you follow advice. A walking book will claim that walking is better than anything else, and so on. But, in fact, it's impossible to make a generalised statement that a certain exercise is better than another because it depends on each individual's specific goal.

Swimming has often been touted as the best all-round exercise. It is well-rounded – you can develop good posture, a firm body and cardiovascular endurance from a low-impact swimming regimen. But if you want to lose weight there is some debate over how much fat is conserved in cold water, so for this purpose it may not be as effective as running or stepping. Or if you have shoulder, neck or back problems, some of the strokes may exacerbate the weakness and cause more pain.

edge in sports can be dangerous. You can't play the sport just to get fit, or you're setting yourself up for an injury. It's better to get fit first in order to play the sport.

So if you aren't the sporty type, you'll probably feel much more comfortable working at your own pace in the uncompetitive club environment. Don't be intimidated into thinking that everybody at a health club is a super-fit hardbody. The majority of health club members are average people trying to get fit. A club environment is slower and more controlled. Since the focus is on fitness first and activity second, there is more emphasis on safe technique and sound alignment. While it's still possible to have an imbalanced workout, there are usually instructors to supervise your general routine. Motivation is hard to muster though, so any variety in a fitness regimen will keep up your interest. And, while they're not ditching their treadmills, many clubs are expanding their repertoires to include outdoor activities. Weekly jogging groups or power-walking sessions are becoming popular. Though a health club may lack vitamin D and panoramic views, the social ambience and encouraging staff may be the best exercise prescription if you want a little prodding. The bottom line is, be open to both choices.

Finding the Right Club for You

Whether you're a club member looking for a change of venue or you've decided to take up a healthy new lifestyle, finding the right place to work out needs investigation. Being faced with chrome, blaring beats and fluorescent lycra can be intimidating. Don't look at what the club has, but at what it can do for you. The personality of the club should suit yours. Before you start looking, identify what you like, what you need, the type of people you associate with, and then find the club that has the closest match.

Most clubs have a distinct atmosphere. If you like intensive workouts you might join a hard-core gym. If you like casual activity that caters for everyone in the family, you might try a local leisure centre. If glitz, glamour and socialising during weight sets is your style, you might try a luxury private health club where high fitness fashion is the standard uniform. Some city clubs have a high proportion of executive members who do a serious workout and then go home; others cater for mothers and provide crèches.

Be aware, however, that your needs may change. The Living Well Health and Leisure Group surveyed the 7000 members of its chain of clubs. While 80 per cent said they joined because there was a pool, after six months only 25 per cent of those members used it regularly. In other words, new members were exposed to activities and equipment they had not considered before. Interestingly enough, men refused to do aerobics when they joined, but six months later many had succumbed to classes designed for them.

A high percentage of the people who join clubs rarely or never use them, and about fifty per cent don't join for a second term. City-centre sites have a higher proportion of people sticking with them; suburban sites tend to have more members who use the facilities very infrequently. To counteract this tendency to quit, choose a club with features that will help you stay. The Living Well survey found that most people stay because of qualified staff and cleanliness. Clubs with the best retention rates are those with the best service.

Some clubs consist of a single aerobics studio while others may offer a fully equipped gym, pool, beauty therapy rooms and squash courts. A leisure centre may provide an even wider range of facilities which include sporting activities as well. You may not need a fully equipped centre if you only want to use the gym. Some centres offer partial membership which you can upgrade later if you wish.

Staff need to be happy and cheerful as well as knowing what they're talking about. And they need to be able to talk to members.

Nothing should be too much effort. A good club has staff who give customers the motivation to stick to a routine and achieve their goals. When you visit a club for the first time, investigate by walking around on your own and asking members if they would recommend it. The best place to get the gossip is in the sauna or steam room.

Convenience

The club should have the equipment, type of and number of classes you require. Some clubs set 15-minute time limits on cardio-vascular equipment during peak hours. If you want to use machines for longer periods during those times, maybe that club is too crowded for you.

Club operating hours should fit in with your schedule. If you join a club close to home, make sure you can go in the early morning or evening, or outside your work hours. If it closes at 9.30 on weekday evenings, find out if this gives you time to leave work, exercise and shower. Peak times may be early mornings, lunchtimes and evenings. Identify the times you are likely to attend and how busy it will be then.

A club should allow a guest to have a free visit to work out and see what the instructors are like. Check out the club both during the day and in the evening to make sure there's not a long queue for equipment, because that can be very annoying.

If you like taking classes, make sure there is a wide range available. You should check to see that distinctions are made between beginner, intermediate and advanced levels. A comprehensive schedule will include the following classes: stretch, conditioning, hi-lo impact, low impact, step, and circuit training. Don't be fooled by fancy names for classes – find out what they consist of. You might also look for speciality classes like yoga or dance.

Most people join clubs in easy reach of home or work. When it's winter and cold and dark, you're more likely to head for the pub instead of the club if it takes too much effort to get there. If you need parking space, is there enough?

Is there adequate locker storage in the changing room? Are all areas kept clean and dry to prevent the spread of germs and viruses. Are blow-driers, towels, soap and shampoo provided? Are the showers group-style or private and which do you prefer? Are there adequate mirrors and dressing tables? Some clubs have separate gyms for women and men. Women's clubs may have equipment with smaller, more comfortable frames designed for women.

Cost

It can be difficult to distinguish between the multitude of payment options – monthly or yearly, on or off peak, and some which even separate the use of facilities. But the service should suit you, the customer, not the club. Many clubs like to set up periodic direct debit payments. The club is ensured a certain amount of capital with little administration, and the member pays without bills and fees for overdue payments accumulating. While a limited contract is often required, if your circumstances change at worst you'll lose the cost of a couple of months rather than the best part of a year. A club should offer some type of freeze policy for serious injuries, illness and the like, but customers should expect to make a bit of a commitment as well. Sometimes a club won't go out of its way to offer you special deals, so ask.

Security

Perhaps the biggest worry, especially when paying a large membership fee, is how financially stable the club is. You've probably heard the horror stories of people showing up to find their club closed, their money gone. Look for tell-tale signs: are things broken or dirty? And the minute you hear someone say lifetime membership, run.

How can you protect yourself? When looking at a club you can contact the Office of Fair Trading and Companies House for any history of unfair practices. But since gossip travels fast, the best way is to speak to existing customers. Ask members if they know anyone who has fallen ill or moved away. Was the club willing to refund their membership subscription? Trade associations encourage high standards from their members, so look for clubs to be members of the FIA, IRSA, IDEA and ACSM.

If you make a mistake in the club you join, unfortunately there's little redress. Legally, a company going into liquidation would treat their members as creditors. But if there's no money, there's no money. If you're lucky, a nearby club will honour the failed memberships in order to attract new clients.

Sarah hated to run but did it anyway because it kept her weight at the level she liked. For a whole year she would force herself to get up every morning and go through the motions. Finally, she stopped. She was reluctant to try anything else because after her laborious experience she decided she hated exercise.

Lesson *There's no use forcing yourself to do something you don't enjoy because you'll eventually give up, defeating the whole purpose of keeping exercise as part of your lifestyle. Try all the different sports, activities and equipment that you can. You may not like one type but go absolutely mad over another.*

Buying Home Exercise Equipment

There are many devices you can use at home, some better than others. Unless you're prepared to spend a lot of money, most home equipment will not be as sturdy or well made as that in your local club. Before buying a product, see if you can borrow one

to use for a few months. If you don't use it as often as you thought you would, it can turn out to be an expensive dust collector.

There are some inexpensive home items which are good to have on rainy days:

- a step
- free weights (ranging from 3-10 pounds)
- elastic resistance bands and tubes
- fitness videos (by certified fitness instructors)

See Appendix B for more details.

Myth

I can't do aerobics because I'm unco-ordinated

False. If you feel unco-ordinated in a class, the chances are it's not you but the instructor who is at fault. Instructors should design exercise patterns around each specific class. If they stick to rigid routines, they may not be as sensitive to your needs as they could be.

No one can instantly pick up an activity if they've never done it before. A highly co-ordinated dancer is not automatically equipped to play football, she must train to do so. Likewise, an aerobics enthusiast is not necessarily a fabulous dancer. You must train your muscles and brain to co-ordinate the specific muscular patterns required by a given movement.

Finding an Aerobics Instructor or Personal Trainer

Forget the days when exercise teachers were merely cheerleaders. Fitness training techniques are constantly being updated by new research in the exercise sciences, so today's instructor should be a qualified health professional. Although flashy outfits, whoops and hollers and loud music may make it *seem* like harmless fun, don't be mistaken: your joints, heart and muscles are in the instructor's hands. Consider the following:

- Is your instructor a professional? Some teachers run classes merely as a hobby, for others it's a career. Whichever category your instructor fits into, she or he should be certified by a respected organisation. Instructors are even more qualified if they hold a degree in one of the sports sciences or in physical education. But look for both: if they have only the degree they could be well-versed in the science, but not the practical aspects. Just because they may have been dancers or top athletes for 15 years, or did physical training in the army, or are masseurs, doctors or actresses, this does not mean that they practice safe, up-to-date techniques. In fact, if that's their only training and they do not hold a current qualification, it might mean the opposite.

- Does the instructor keep up to date with skills and new research? Some qualify and then never bother learning anything again. At the time of publishing, the standard British qualification, the RSA certificate, does not require renewal so instructors may not have continued their education. Make sure that your instructor regularly attends training workshops and national and international fitness conventions sponsored by Fitness Professionals, IDEA, AFAA or the Exercise Association (formerly ASSET). It's a good sign too if you see instructors taking part in other teachers' classes. In any profession, continuing education and growth are the key to success.

- Does your instructor stare into the mirror throughout the class? Big egos are usually bad news. Teachers should face the class and focus on you as much as possible.

- Does your teacher count and count and count? Check out the teaching skills: a good teacher *teaches*. On some fitness videos incessant counting wastes valuable time that could be used for instructing, giving explanations and pointing out the intricacies involved with every move.

- Look at Chapter 16, which lists some of the standard stressful moves to avoid. If your teacher includes these, change teachers.

- Gym and class instructors should hold recognised qualifications such as a degree in exercise science, PE or dance. They should also be certified by one or more of the following:

  The American Council on Exercise (ACE)

  The European Fitness Instructor Certification (EFIC)

  The Aerobics & Fitness Association of America (AFAA)

  RSA (plus regularly attend continuing education)

  The Physical Education Association (PEA)

  The American College of Sports Medicine (ACSM)

  The Australian Council for Health, Physical Education and Recreation

Perform the warm-up stretches in Chapter 16 and begin your chosen programme. Don't forget to read the last four chapters to find out how to stay motivated.

PART THREE

THE BODY TRANSFORMATION CURVES

Now that you have learned exactly what you need to do, you can follow your chosen Body Transformation Curve.

Each Curve consists of a 12-week progressive exercise programme. These Curves include basic activities such as walking, aerobics classes, swimming and conditioning exercises. You may follow these as they are, or personalise your plan by substituting some of the activities on your final list (Chapter 10). Whenever possible, try to substitute activities of similar impact and intensity. See the beginning of section 2 if you'd like to be reminded of the different Curves you can follow. You may use the blank schedules provided to write down your substitute activities.

Before you start your curve, use the stretch exercises which follow to warm up.

Week	Mon	Tues	Wed	Thurs	Fri	Sat	Sun
1							
2							
3							
4							
5							
6							
7							
8							
9							
10							
11							
12							

Stretch

No matter which Curve you choose to follow, it's a good idea to begin and end each exercise session with a short series of stretches and warming up/cooling down moves. You may attend a fitness class, watch a video or follow the exercises I demonstrate for you here.

WARMING UP

Research has shown that your muscles will respond better to exercise if you prepare them first by slowly easing them into a more intense workload. As you do this, your joints will become lubricated and other bodily changes take place so that your exercise session functions as efficiently as possible.

There is no one set way to warm up. Generally, the easiest thing to do is to start your chosen activity very slowly. If you are going running, start by walking for about five minutes. If you are going cycling, start by cycling very slowly for five minutes. If you are playing a sport or taking a fitness class your warm-up could be as simple as marching or walking on the spot while simulating some of the arm movements you'll use in the activity later on.

Warm up for about 5–10 minutes before you begin any exercise. This will get the blood flowing, the joints lubricated and the muscles prepared for more intense activity. March on the spot or walk slowly, adding simple arm movements at various intervals. Follow your warm-up with some slow, static (on the spot) stretches (see below).

STRETCHING

The following stretches target most of the key muscle groups you'll be using. There is no research to prove that stretching will decrease your chances of injury, but it *will* help your body feel better – looser and more agile – as you move. Try to do these stretches

---

Myth

To increase flexibility, you should stretch as far as possible

False. It is common for some people to bounce and force the muscles to stretch even further than normal. These two practices actually counteract the purpose of stretching (to relax and lengthen) by activating the stretch reflex. A muscle fibre will contract when it senses it is about to be overstretched. So bouncing or forcing a stretch can result in microtears in the muscle fibres. Pain is a good indicator of how to stretch. If it hurts, stop. Stretches should be static (still) in order to *coax* rather than *force* the muscles into lengthening. Stretching also releases endorphins (which are also released during orgasm, so the stretch should always feel good!).

for five minutes or so before and after your workout. The American College of Sports Medicine recommends that you do flexibility exercises for 30 minutes at least twice a week. If you miss a session, it probably won't hurt, but the stretches are a good way to start and

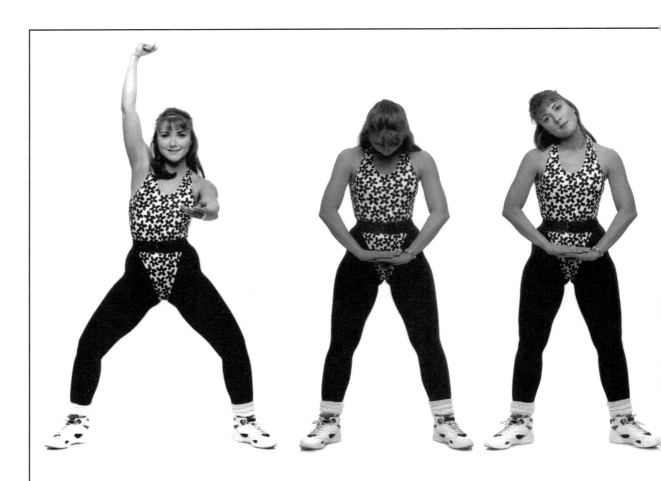

1. Torso Stretch

Stand with your legs in a straddle position, feet shoulder-width apart. Keep your knees slightly bent and reach your left arm away from your chest while lifting your right arm to the ceiling. Concentrate on lifting your ribs away from your hips to lengthen your spine. Hold the stretch until you feel your muscles relax. Switch sides.

2. Neck Stretch

Clasp your hands in front of your body. Hold your ribs up shoulders down. Gently allow your head to drop towards your chest. Hold until you feel some of the tension release from the muscles in the back of your neck.

Now, keep your torso lifted, but relaxed. Drop your right ear to your right shoulder. Hold for five seconds then carefully allow your head to roll forward to the other shoulder.

end your workouts. Hold each stretch for 10–30 seconds.

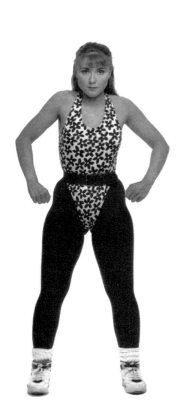
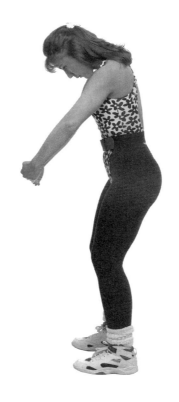
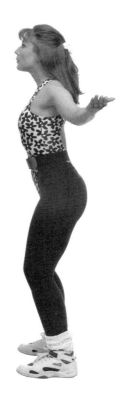

3. Shoulder Circles

Circle your shoulders forward very slowly four times. Reverse.

4. Upper Back Stretch

Clasp your hands in front of your body. Drop your chin and round your shoulders forward so you feel a stretch in the middle of your upper back. Hold.

5. Chest Stretch

Rotate your palms out and open your arms to the side. Press your chest forward.

71

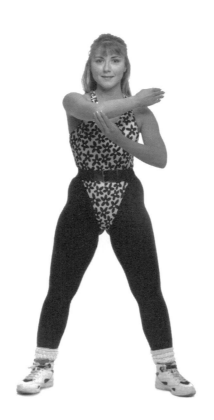 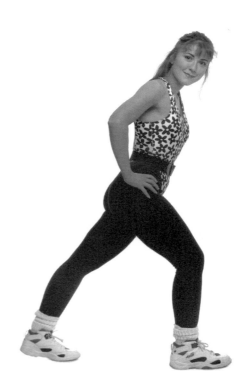

6. Shoulder Stretch

Gently press your right elbow towards the opposite shoulder. Hold, then switch sides.

7. Hip and Thigh Stretch

Stand with your feet wide apart, your right leg in front of your body, the left back. Make sure both toes point forward. Press your left hip forward so you feel a stretch in the area where your pelvis and upper thigh connect. When these muscles release, bend your left knee slightly so you feel a stretch in the front of your left thigh. If you feel pain in your left knee, straighten your leg more. Switch sides.

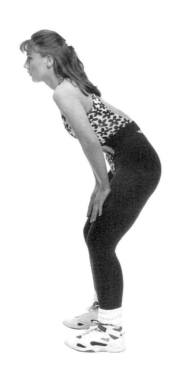
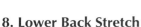
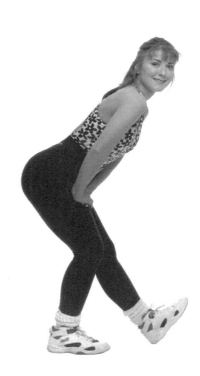
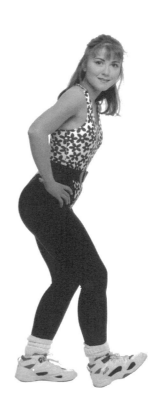

8. Lower Back Stretch

Stand in a straddle position with your knees slightly bent. Lean forward at an angle and support the weight of your torso by resting your hands on your thighs. Press your chest forward. Hold, then contract your abdominals and round your lower back.

9. Back of the Thigh and Calf Stretch

Place your right leg slightly in front of your body. Bend your left leg and support the weight of your torso on your back leg as you lean forward. Push backward with your tailbone. Start with your front toe down then, as you feel the muscle in the back of your leg loosen up, lift your toe. If this hurts your calf too much, lower your toe slightly. Hold.

10. Front and Back of Calf Stretch

Place your right leg slightly in front of your body. Bend your left leg and support the weight of your torso on your back leg as you lean forward. Bend your front knee a little and lift and lower your toe repeatedly. This warms up the muscles in the front of your lower leg. Then hold your toe up to feel a stretch in your calf.

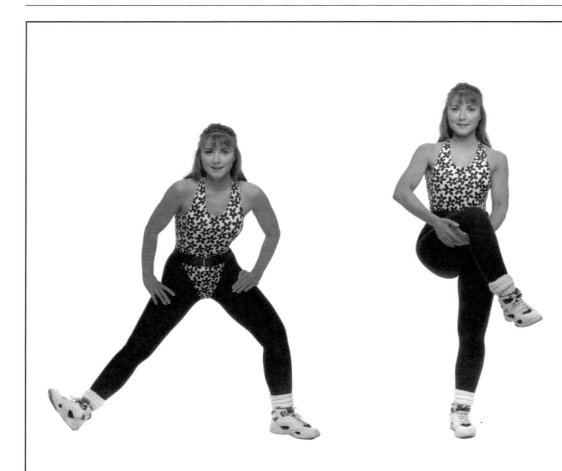

11. Inner Thigh Stretch

Stand in a wide straddle position and support both hands on your thighs. Bend your left knee and straighten your right leg. Make sure your legs are wide enough apart so that your left knee stops above your ankle, not your toe. Hold the stretch until your inner thighs relax, then switch sides.

12. Gluteals Stretch

Stand with your knees slightly bent. Slowly bend your right knee and hold it to your chest. You may wish to place your right hand on a chair or wall for balance. Cross your thighs over towards the other side. Hold, then switch legs.

COOLING DOWN

Slow down gradually after an intense exercise session. For example, if you're running, bring it down to a walk. If you're stepping on a bench, step on the floor. Stopping abruptly causes lactic acid to build up in the muscle which can then leads to soreness. You can also become dizzy.

Slow the movements down until your heart rate returns to normal, or about 100 beats per minute. Finish with some more slow stretches, targeting the muscles you have just worked. A proper cool-down and stretch should make you feel relaxed and energised.

Myth

**Waist exercises such as twisting and bending from
side to side will result in inches off your waist**

These exercises have been incorporated into some classes and touted as being waist slimmers. They are not. At worst, the rapid repetition of waist twists and bends has the potential to damage the spinal discs and associated ligaments. Physiologists advise that to decrease fat from the torso and waist area, you must carry out regular aerobic exercise (cycling, running, rowing, aerobic dance, etc). These activities will burn fat from all over the body. Also recommended to help strengthen the abdominal muscles are half sit-ups (crunches) and lifting up and rotating slightly to the side

Avoid These Risky Exercises

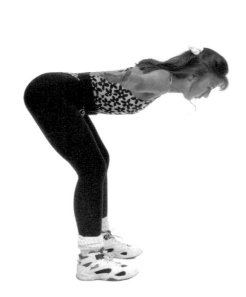
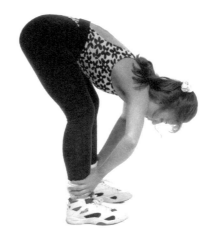

1. Flat back, touching toes

Although you probably did this for years in gym class, research has shown that bending forward with an unsupported back can compress the discs between your vertebrae and strain the spinal ligaments.

Traditionally, these stretches have been used to stretch the back of the *thighs*, *not* the back. A safer alternative, then, is to do stretch number 9 (Back of the Thigh and Calf Stretch) or a lying-down hamstring stretch.

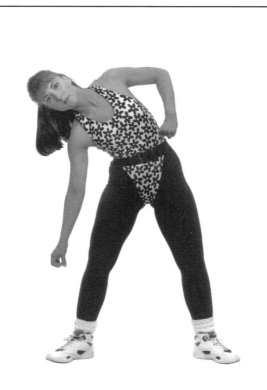

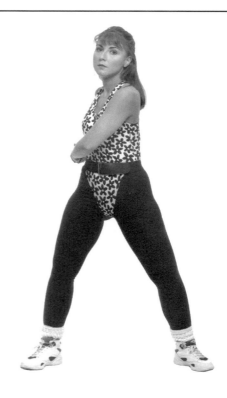

2. Deep side bends/twists

Lots of unqualified fitness gurus have twisted and bent for years, claiming that this move will help trim your waist. In fact, all it could do is strain your spine. To target the waist you need to do abdominal exercises to acquire muscle tone and high calorie-burning activities to get rid of excess fat. To stretch the waist try stretch number 1 (Torso Stretch).

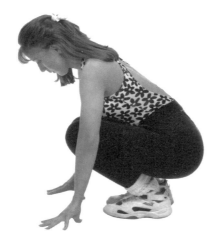

3. Deep knee bends

This position puts lots of strain on the ligaments in the front of your knees. It can stretch your calves, but there are better ways to do so without stressing the knees. Try stretch number 10 (Front and Back of Calf Stretch).

Myth

**Bending forward from the waist while standing or
sitting is a good way to stretch your body**

False. This position, called forward flexion, is potentially unsafe. It can overstretch supportive back ligaments which might never regain their original elasticity. It can also compress one side of the intervertebral discs causing the other side to bulge. In addition, this position increases the risk of a ruptured spinal disc.

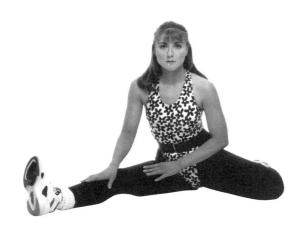 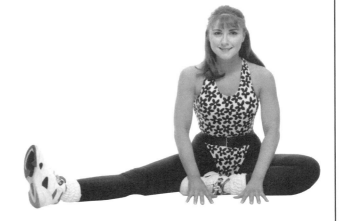

4. Hurdler stretch

Instead bend the foot in

This position looks harmless except that the knee is twisted precariously. Since the knee is a hinge joint (as on a door), it bends front and back, but is not designed to twist. Twisting the knee can overstretch some knee ligaments or strain other structures in the knee joint. For a safer inner thigh stretch, remain seated in this position, but bend your foot in, rather than out.

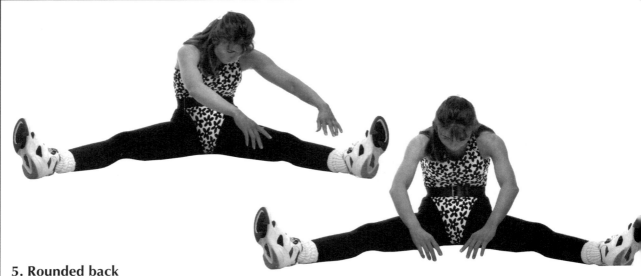

5. Rounded back

Since it's very likely that you slouch at your desk or in chairs, excessive forward bending of the spine can put it at risk. Instead of trying to touch your thighs by rounding your back, aim to keep a straight back and just lean slightly forward. In this stretch of the back or inner

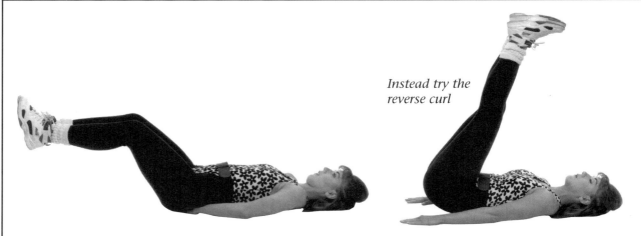

Instead try the reverse curl

6. Double leg lift

Many people are under the impression that this is a great exercise to strengthen your abdominals. In fact what makes this exercise tough is the extremely excessive stress on your lower back as it arches to try to balance your body when your legs are lifted. And the muscle burns you feel are not the abdominals but small muscles in the front of the hips called the hip flexors. Since you probably strengthen your hip flexors enough if you step, cycle, or even walk, making them too strong can adversely affect your lower back.

To target the abdominals instead of these other areas, just bring your legs closer to your body as demonstrated in the Reverse Curl. Keep them there and, instead of moving your legs up and down, just tilt your pelvis slightly.

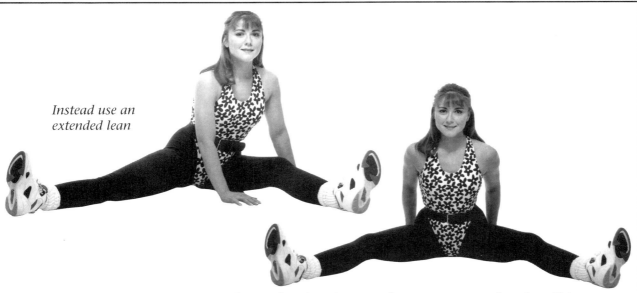

Instead use an extended lean

thighs, it is unnecessary to go right to the floor. As long as you feel a pleasant stretch-ing in your leg, you are performing this move correctly.

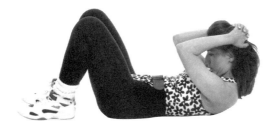

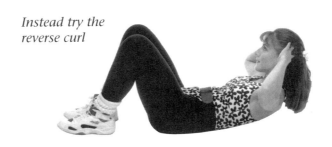

Instead try the reverse curl

7. Pulling on the head/full sit-up

Sit-ups are done to work the abdominal muscles. This is achieved by lifting your chest up to a 45° angle off the floor. When you lift higher than that other muscles in your hips take over the work. The amount of force needed to lift the body high and rapidly usually means that the neck ends up being pulled and strain-ed. It's more effective to do a half sit-up, or crunch.

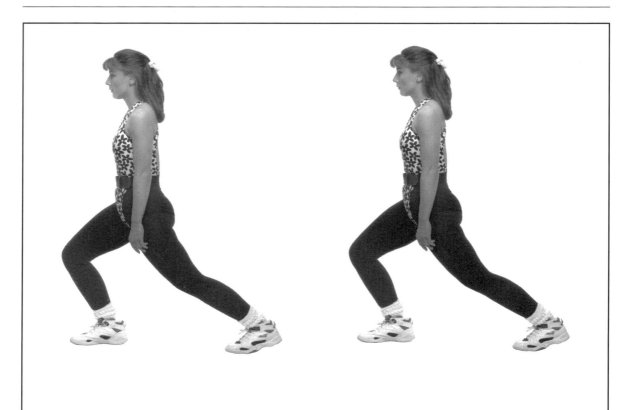

8. Acute lunge

Whenever your legs are close together and you bend your knees, there is a tendency for the knees to jut forward past your toes. This can put too much stress on ligaments in the front of your knees. For a safer, and sturdier, position, open your legs very wide and bend your knee so that it remains above your ankles, not your toes. Make sure your calf is perpendicular to the floor, not slanted.

Instead try the square lunge

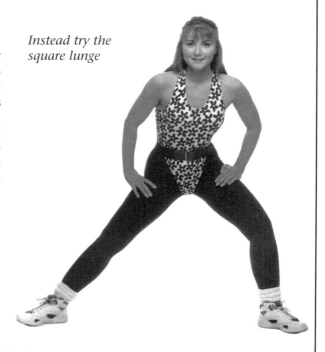

CHAPTER 13

The Health Curve

IMPROVE YOUR OVERALL HEALTH; DECREASE YOUR RISK OF LONG-TERM DISEASES.

This programme will focus on frequent bouts of low-intensity exercise – walking or walking to the shops, swimming, biking and gardening. Remember, you can substitute some of the activities for those on your list, but the key is to introduce as much 'easy' activity into everyday life as possible. It includes one day a week of conditioning exercises to preserve the structural integrity of your joints, and allows for rest days. The idea is to be relatively active and not worry too much about how hard you're working. Feel free to break up the day's workouts so that the requirement is fulfilled in several shorter blocks.

Week	Mon	Tues	Wed	Thurs	Fri	Sat	Sun
1							
2							
3							
4							
5							
6							
7							
8							
9							
10							
11							
12							

There are only two levels because you should achieve benefits without having to do advanced levels of activity.

Progress at your own pace. Listen to your body. If the increases in intensity or duration are too much for you on a particular day or week, go back to the schedule for the previous week. If an activity is inconvenient or not to your liking, look at your list and substitute one of a similar intensity and the same or lesser impact and include it on the blank schedule on page 81.

Identify your current fitness level	Follow:
You haven't exercised or done any aerobic activities for more than six months	Level One
You exercise sporadically (walk, run, dance)	Level Two

Notes: All figures indicate the number of minutes. c = conditioning exercises (see **Conditioning for Curves** in Chapter 17). These should be undertaken where indicated *in addition* to the other activity specified for that day. You won't start conditioning exercises until you've built up a bit of strength after two weeks. Walk to and from the shops for a time totalling at least 30 minutes (15 each way).

LEVEL ONE

Week	Mon	Tues	Wed	Thurs	Fri	Sat	Sun
1	walk 10				bike 10	garden 30	
2	bike 10		walk 15			walk shops	garden 30
3	bike 12		swim 10	walk 20 c		garden 30	
4	bike 12		swim 12 c	walk 20			garden 30
5	swim 15	walk 20		bike 15 c		garden 30	
6	walk 25		bike 15 c	swim 15		walk shops	garden 30
7	walk 30		swim 18	walk 30 c		garden 30	swim 18
8	walk 30		bike 20		swim 20 c	walk shops	garden 30
9	walk 20 c	walk 30		bike 20	walk 30	garden 30	
10	walk 30		swim 20 c	bike 25		walk shops	garden 30
11	swim 20	walk 30		bike 25 c		bike 25	garden 30
12	walk 30		walk 30 c		swim 20	walk shops	garden 30

LEVEL TWO

Week	Mon	Tues	Wed	Thurs	Fri	Sat	Sun
1	walk 20		walk 20 c		bike 15	garden 30	
2	bike 15		walk 20	bike 15 c		walk shops	garden 30
3	bike 20		swim 15 c	walk 25		garden 30	walk 25
4	bike 20		swim 15	walk 25	walk 25 c		garden 30
5	swim 20	walk 30	bike 25 c			garden 30	swim 20
6	walk 30		bike 25	swim 25 c		walk shops	garden 30
7			walk 30	swim 25 c	walk 30		garden 30
8	walk 30		bike 25		swim 20 c	walk shops	garden 30
9		swim 25	walk 30 c		bike 30	walk 30	garden 30
10	walk 30		swim 25	bike 30 c		walk shops	garden 30
11	swim 30	walk 30		bike 30		bike 30 c	garden 30
12	walk 30		walk 30 c		swim 20	walk shops	garden 30

Joanne was used to walking to and from the bus stop every day on the way to work. It took about 15 minutes each way. When she got a new car she was able to drive to work, and a year later she noticed she had gained 15 pounds. She was eating the same amount and did not do any formal exercise, but then she never had. So she consulted a personal trainer and together they worked out that the 30 minutes of walking she had previously done five days a week used up a total of 52,000 calories over the course of a year – calories she was now no longer using up. One pound in weight equals about 3500 calories. Using this same calculation, it's easy to see that Joanne's excess 15 pounds could largely be attributed to the 52,000 calories she was no longer burning.

Lesson *Even informal exercise uses calories. If you don't have time to work out every day, using the stairs instead of the lift or getting off the bus a stop or two early and walking the rest of the way can add up over a period of time.*

CHAPTER 14

The Energy Curve

IMPROVE YOUR ENDURANCE/STAMINA; INCREASE YOUR ENERGY LEVELS AND ABILITY TO DO EVERYDAY ACTIVITIES SUCH AS CLIMBING STAIRS.

The Energy Curve is designed to get your major systems back into smooth running order. The aerobic element will increase your stamina, the anaerobic element will provide you with quick energy, and the muscle-conditioning exercises will keep your body strong.

There are only two levels because you should achieve benefits without having to do advanced levels of activity.

Remember to progress at your own pace. Listen to your body. If the increases in intensity or duration are too much for you on a

Week	Mon	Tues	Wed	Thurs	Fri	Sat	Sun
1							
2							
3							
4							
5							
6							
7							
8							
9							
10							
11							
12							

particular day or week, go back to the schedule for the previous week. If an activity is inconvenient or not to your liking, look at your list and substitute one of a similar intensity and the same or lesser impact and include it on the blank schedule opposite. If you wish, you may substitute something of higher impact and intensity, in which case you may reduce the time spent exercising by about fifty per cent.

Identify your current fitness level	Follow:
You haven't exercised or done any aerobic activities for more than six months	Level One
You exercise sporadically (walk, run, dance)	Level Two

Notes: All figures indicate the number of minutes.   c = conditioning exercises; cr = conditioning exercises with added resistance (see **Conditioning for Curves** in Chapter 17). These should be undertaken where indicated *in addition* to the other activity specified for that day.

LEVEL ONE

Week	Mon	Tues	Wed	Thurs	Fri	Sat	Sun
1	walk 15		walk 15		bike 15 c		
2	bike 15		walk 15 c	bike 15		step 15 c	
3	bike 20	step 15 c	walk 20		walk 20		
4	bike 20		step 20 cr	walk 25	walk 25 c		
5	step 20	walk 25 cr		bike 25 cr		step 20	
6	walk 25 cr		bike 20	step 25 cr	walk 25		
7	walk 30 cr		step 25	walk 30 cr	swim 15	bike 20	
8	walk 30 cr		bike 20	walk 35 cr	step 20	swim 15	
9		swim 15	walk 30 c		step 20	walk 30 c	bike 25
10	walk 30 c		swim 15	bike 25 c	step 20		walk 35
11	swim 20 c		bike 25	step 20 c		walk 35	step 20
12		walk 35 c	swim 20		walk 40 c	bike 30	step 25

LEVEL TWO

Week	Mon	Tues	Wed	Thurs	Fri	Sat	Sun
1	walk 30		walk 30 c		bike 20	swim 20 c	
2	bike 20		walk 30 c	bike 20		swim 20 c	
3	bike 25		step 15 c	walk 35		walk 35 c	
4	bike 25 c	walk 35		step 15 cr	swim 25	walk 35	
5	step 20	walk 35 cr		bike 25 cr	step 20		walk 35
6	walk 40 cr		bike 30	step 25 cr	walk 40		swim 25
7	walk 40 cr	step 25	walk 45 cr		step 25	swim 30	
8	walk 40 cr		bike 20	walk 40 cr	step 25		swim 30
9	walk 45	step 30 c		bike 25	walk 45 c		swim 30
10		walk 50 c	bike 25		step 30	walk 50 c	swim 35
11	walk 55		bike 30 c	step 35	walk 55 c		swim 35
12		walk 60 c	bike 30		step 35	swim 40 c	bike 35

Should you exercise when you're tired?

We all need different amounts of sleep (between seven and nine hours is the average). If you regularly make do with less than five hours, it could start to show physically and mentally.

While exercise can wake you up if you just need a jump start, it can also slow you down if what you really need is rest. Don't be afraid to take a day off. Rest is as important as exercise.

CHAPTER 15

The Body Curve

LOSE WEIGHT OR BODY FAT, RESCULPT YOUR BODY; IMPROVE STRENGTH AND MUSCLE TONE.

To lose fat and reshape your body you need to burn enough calories and develop enough muscle mass so that you use up fat stores while building a firm body. If you are fairly fit already and not overweight then you may wish to concentrate on more intense muscle-conditioning work. If you are overweight your emphasis should primarily be on using up calories, in which case you may want to do more aerobic work than conditioning. The exercise should be performed at as high an intensity as you can work out safely. The lower the intensity, the longer you'll need to work out so you can burn the greatest number of

Week	Mon	Tues	Wed	Thurs	Fri	Sat	Sun
1							
2							
3							
4							
5							
6							
7							
8							
9							
10							
11							
12							

calories.

For best results eat a low-fat diet. Your caloric intake should not be lower than 1200 calories per day. Aim for weight loss of no more than 2 pounds (1 kg) per week.

Here, I ask you to undertake some conditioning exercise two or three times a week. Use free weights, weight machines or elastic bands. Aim for one or two sets of 8–12 repetitions.

The Body Curve has three levels. Remember to progress at your own pace. Listen to your body. If the increases in intensity or duration are too much for you on a particular day or week, go back to the schedule for the previous week. If an activity is inconvenient or not to your liking, substitute an activity from your list for one of a similar intensity and the same or lesser impact and include it on the blank schedule on page 87.

Notes: All figures indicate the number of minutes. c = conditioning exercises; cr = conditioning exercises with added resistance (see **Conditioning for Curves** in Chapter 17). These should be undertaken where indicated *in addition* to the other activity specified for that day. step/aer = take a step class or aerobics class. step/li = take a step or low impact class or video. bike/aer = bike or take an aerobics class or video. walk/jog = walk or jog or do a mixture of both. sm = stairmaster or stairclimber machine.

LEVEL ONE

Week	Mon	Tues	Wed	Thurs	Fri	Sat	Sun
1	walk 10	walk 15 c		bike 10			
2	bike 10		walk 15 c	bike 12			walk 15
3	bike 12		step 10 c	walk 20		walk 20 c	
4	bike 12		step 12 cr	walk 20	walk 23	bike 15 cr	
5	step 15	walk 23 cr		bike 15 cr		walk 25 cr	step 15
6	walk 25 cr		bike 15		step 15 cr	walk 25	bike 18 cr
7	walk 30 cr		step 18	walk 30 cr		bike 18 cr	step 18
8	walk 35 cr		bike 20	walk 35 cr		step 20	walk 35 cr
9		step 20	walk 40 cr		bike 20 cr	walk 40	step 20
10	walk 40 cr		step 20 cr	bike 22		step 25 cr	walk 40
11	bike 25 cr		walk 40 cr	bike 25		step 25	walk 45
12		step 25 cr	walk 45		bike 25 cr	walk 45	step 25 cr

Identify your current fitness level	Follow:
You haven't exercised or done any aerobic activities for more than six months	Level One
You exercise sporadically (walk, run, dance)	Level Two
You are a regular exerciser but looking for a change or trying to overcome a plateau	Level Three

Myth

Exercise makes me eat more, so it defeats the purpose of exercising

False. Low to moderate amounts of exercise actually suppress the appetite in most people. Very intense exercise does increase the appetite, but usually the person does not consume as many calories as they have used, so there is still a positive effect on weight loss.

LEVEL TWO

Week	Mon	Tues	Wed	Thurs	Fri	Sat	Sun
1	walk 25	bike 20 c		step 20		walk 25 c	bike 20
2	walk 30		step 20 c	bike 20		walk 30 c	step 20
3	walk 35 c		step/aer 30		bike 25 cr	walk 20	bike 25 cr
4		walk/jog 35 cr	step/li 25		bike 25 cr	walk/jog 25	bike 25 cr
5		step 25 cr	walk/jog 35/ aer 25 cr	bike 25 cr	step/aer 25	walk 40 cr	
6		walk 35 cr	bike/aer 30	walk 40 cr		step/aer 30	bike 30 cr
7	walk 40/ aer 30		step 30 cr	bike/aer 30		walk 35 cr	bike 30 cr
8	walk 40/ aer 30	bike 35 cr		walk 35 cr		step/aer 30	bike 35 cr
9	walk 45 cr	step/aer 30	bike 35 cr		run 15 cr	step/aer 30	
10		walk 45 cr	run 15	bike 40 cr		walk 50	run 15 cr
11		bike 45 cr	walk 50 cr	run 20	bike 45 cr		step/aer 30
12		walk 55 cr	run 20	bike 45 cr		run 25 cr	swim 20

Melissa had been plump all her life but had a pretty face so never became too obsessed about it. When she finally decided she wanted to lose weight she started walking *occasionally* but her weight didn't change much.

Lesson *She had done virtually no activity all her life and the small amount she started to do was so sporadic that it didn't do much in the way of weight loss. If you want to see results your activity must be fairly rigorous consistent.*

LEVEL THREE

Week	Mon	Tues	Wed	Thurs	Fri	Sat	Sun
1	walk 60 cr	bike 30/step 20		run 30	swim 25 cr		walk 60
2	bike 30/step 20 cr	aer/run 30		swim 25 cr	walk 60	aer/run 30 cr	swim 25
3		walk 65 cr	bike 35/sm 25	aer/run 35 cr		swim 30	bike 35 cr
4		step class cr	swim 30	run 40 cr		run 40 cr	
5	walk 65		step/aer cr	bike 40	swim 30 cr	walk 65	run 35 cr
6		bike 40 cr	swim 35		walk 65 cr	step/sm 25	run 40 cr
7	swim 40		step/aer cr	bike 45	walk 65 cr		run 45 cr
8	swim 40	bike 45 cr	step/aer		run 45 cr	bike 45/sm 25	walk 65 cr
9	run 45	bike 45 cr		run 45 cr	step/aer		walk 65 cr
10	run 50	bike 50 cr		swim 45 cr	walk 65	bike 50 cr	
11	step/aer cr		run 50	bike 50 cr		walk 65 cr	run 50
12	walk 65 cr	swim 50		step/aer cr		run 55	bike 55 cr

CHAPTER 16

The Serenity Curve

REDUCE STRESS; IMPROVE YOUR MENTAL WELL–BEING.

The Serenity Curve includes some aerobic work such as walking and swimming which will help your mind deal with stress. It also includes some `thinking' exercise such as yoga and Pilates techniques which will help you learn to distance yourself from your problems so that they can be seen in a healthier, larger perspective. Use the visualisation given at the end of this chapter for your own meditation and relaxation.

Some flexibility stretches are included at least twice a week to help release muscular tension (see Chapter 12 for guidelines). They should be performed slowly, working towards a greater range of motion in the joint. Hold each stretch for 10–30 seconds.

Week	Mon	Tues	Wed	Thurs	Fri	Sat	Sun
1							
2							
3							
4							
5							
6							
7							
8							
9							
10							
11							
12							

Do 3–5 repetitions of each exercise. Do not stretch so far that you feel pain. If you choose to do yoga, Pilates or one of the martial arts, please be aware that some of the movements can stress your lower back and knees (see Chapter 12). Avoid these.

There are only two levels because you should achieve benefits without having to do advanced levels of activity.

Remember to progress at your own pace. Listen to your body. If the increases in intensity or duration are too much for you on a particular day or week, go back to the schedule for the previous week. If an activity is inconvenient or not to your liking, substitute one from your list of a similar intensity and the same or lesser impact, and include it on the blank schedule on page 91.

Note: All figures indicate the number of minutes. Yoga: you may take a yoga class at your local health club or leisure centre or try a reputable video. See Chapter 12 for stretching exercises. You can be flexible in the time you spend on yoga and meditation

LEVEL ONE

Week	Mon	Tues	Wed	Thurs	Fri	Sat	Sun
1	walk 15	stretch15		meditate 15		yoga	
2	stretch 15		walk 15		meditate		swim 15
3	yoga		walk 20	meditate	stretch 15		swim 15
4	walk 20	meditate	stretch 20		yoga		swim 15
5	meditate	walk 20		stretch 20	swim 20		yoga
6	6	swim 20		stretch 20		walk 20	yoga
7	meditate	walk 25	yoga		swim 20		stretch 25
8	walk 25		yoga		stretch 25	meditate	swim 20
9	meditate	walk 25	stretch 25		swim 25		yoga
10	walk 30		yoga		stretch 25	meditate	swim 20
11	yoga	walk 30		stretch 30	meditate	swim 25	
12	walk 30		yoga	swim 25	meditate	stretch 30	

Identify your current fitness level	Follow:
You haven't exercised or done any aerobic activities for more than six months	Level One
You are a regular exerciser but looking to make your workout less frenzied, more peaceful	Level Two

Meditation

Meditation is simply the act of clearing the mind and focusing on one thing. By relaxing your mind your body will also relax. Your breath will become slow and deep.

In the beginning it can be quite difficult to meditate for long periods of time. The mind is easily distracted. It takes training to be able to focus only on your breathing, or a word, or a thought. You can meditate by just controlling your breathing. Breathe in slowly through your nose for a count of four. Hold

LEVEL TWO

Week	Mon	Tues	Wed	Thurs	Fri	Sat	Sun
1	walk 20	meditate	stretch 20	Pilates		yoga	walk 30
2	meditate	walk 25	yoga		swim 20	stretch 20	walk 25
3	yoga		walk 30	swim 25	meditate	Pilates	walk 30
4	Pilates	walk 30		stretch 25	swim 25		yoga
5	walk 35	Pilates		yoga	swim 25	meditate	stretch 30
6	walk 35	yoga		swim 30	stretch 30	meditate	Pilates 30
7	meditate	walk 35	swim 30		Pilates	stretch 30	walk 35
8	meditate	swim 30	yoga	walk 35		Pilates	stretch 30
9	walk 40	yoga	meditate	Pilates		swim 30	stretch 30
10	yoga	walk 40	Pilates		stretch 30	meditate	swim 30
11	walk 45	stretch 30	meditate	yoga		Pilates	swim 30
12	yoga	walk 45		Pilates	meditate	swim 30	stretch 30

your breath for a count of two, then exhale slowly from your nose for a count of six. After you have established a rhythmic breathing pattern you can focus on relaxing different areas of your body, or visualising a positive image to inspire or relax you. You may also breathe in different patterns, but it's best to seek advice from a yoga or meditation expert.

In the beginning aim to meditate for five minutes. As you progress over the weeks you can gradually add more time. You'll be surprised at how good you feel after just five or ten minutes.

Here is a meditation you can use to help you relax. You may wish to read it into a tape recorder in a slow, calm, soothing voice. Then play it back while you are lying down in a quiet place. Turn off the phone, close your door and make your environment as comfortable as possible.

Serenity Meditation

- Lie on your back with your arms and legs straight. Close your eyes and begin breathing very slowly. When you inhale, breathe the air through the back of your nostrils with as little physical effort as possible. Let the air fill up the bottom of your lungs first, then the middle, then the top. Feel your lungs expanding like a balloon. Let the air soak in for a few seconds then slowly exhale, again through the back of the nostrils. Empty the air first from the bottom, then from the middle, then from the top of your lungs. Keep your lungs empty and relaxed for one second, then slowly begin the rhythmic wave of breathing again.

- Remember you are in no hurry to breathe. Pause before you inhale and before you exhale. You are luxuriating in every oxygen molecule that enters your body. Continue to breathe and notice how the focus on your breath brings you inwards to a peaceful, calm place. As you inhale notice the rise of your ribcage. Feel your lungs expand. As you exhale notice your chest fall; feel your lungs deflate. Continue to breathe as slowly as you can. Slowly in and slowly out until the slow wave becomes automatic, the air gliding effortlessly in, and out, of your nose.

- When you have settled into a calm resting state, continue breathing in this same pattern. But now bring the focus to your eyes. Make them soft. Unclench your eyebrows. Smooth out the lines in your forehead. Every time you breathe out you can feel the tension sliding down the sides of your face, leaving it smooth and unrippled.

- Your lips are together, but your teeth are apart. Relax your tongue to the bottom of your mouth. Feel the back of your head sinking into the floor. Your neck is relaxed.

- Bring your focus gently down your torso, down your legs, to your feet. Continue breathing slowly. As you exhale relax your toes. Allow your feet to fall naturally. Feel that they are supported, but with no effort from you.

- Still breathing slowly in, slowly out bring the focus to your thighs.

- Your knees are soft, not locked. Your thighs are unclenched and slightly rotated to the side as they have fallen into a relaxed state.

- Keep your buttocks soft, allow your lower back to sink into the floor.

- As you exhale, travel with your mind up from the base of your spine to the middle. Still breathing deeply, continue up and focus on the area between the shoulder blades. Imagine tight knotted muscles which are forcing your shoulder blades close together. With each subsequent exhalation allow those knots to disappear, to melt. So that your shoulder blades gradually ease away from each other and sink into the floor.

- Focus on the area between your shoulders and neck. If your shoulders are clenched, let them flop down, relax.
- Still breathing slowly in, slowly out, travel.

- With your mind down each arm. Relax your fingers. Allow your hands to rest where they lie.

- Still breathing deeply, pause before you inhale, pause before you exhale.

- Your toes, tongue and forehead are relaxed. Your entire body is relaxed. Notice the peace you feel in this relaxed state. If day-to-day worries or insignificant thoughts keep popping into your mind, gently nudge them away by bringing your focus back to the breath going in and out of your nose, feel the chest rise and fall.

- Continue breathing slowly and imagine yourself being slowly filled with white light. It is entering from the top of your head and slowly seeping, seeping, seeping, with each breath, to the deepest crevices in your body, between tissues, around bones. Filling up your feet, your ankles, your calves, your thighs, your pelvis, your abdomen, your ribcage, your lungs, your neck and shoulders; overflowing into each arm – the fingers, wrist, elbow – andfilling up the entire body so it rises to your head. The warm white light is permeating through your tissues infusing good thoughts and good feelings into your body, into your mind. Continue to breathe as slowly as you can. Imagine yourself bathed in goodness, in white protective light. Relax and continue breathing deeply until you are ready to open your eyes, refreshed and revitalised.

CHAPTER 17

Conditioning for Curves

Once you begin following one of the Body Transformation Curves, you may notice that on several days each week you are instructed to do conditioning exercises (c), or conditioning exercises with resistance (cr). These should be exercises that target the major muscles in your upper and lower body. You may attend body-shaping classes, follow a video or do the following exercises which I demonstrate in this chapter.

The following conditioning movements will help you tone and strengthen specific muscles in your arms, back, chest, hips and thighs. If you are a beginner, perform these exercises *without* resistance (weights) at first. Once you feel that you can accomplish each set of exercises easily, increase the resistance by adding a light weight so you continue to overload, or challenge your muscles.

If you are used to doing many of these exercises, you should probably start using light resistance from the beginning. Start with a weight that is between 1 and 3 lbs.

You should aim to do at least one set of 8-12 repetitions. If you cannot complete the entire number of repetitions, use a lighter weight. If you complete 12 and do not feel fatigued in the muscle you are working, increase the weight. Once you can complete one set, do an additional set until you work up to three full sets. When these become easy, increase the weight slightly.

Certain muscles are stronger than others so you may find that you will need to vary the weight you use for each exercise. If you have just one set of weights you can double them up if you need more weight. See Appendix B for retailers of good-quality resistance equipment.

You may wish to review Chapter 4 on Muscles. Since the muscles you work need time to heal and strengthen, you are better off doing these exercises every other day rather than every day. You should notice your body becoming firmer and stronger in as little as three to four weeks after you begin to follow the exercises.

YOUR UPPER BODY

1. Upper Back (trapezius)

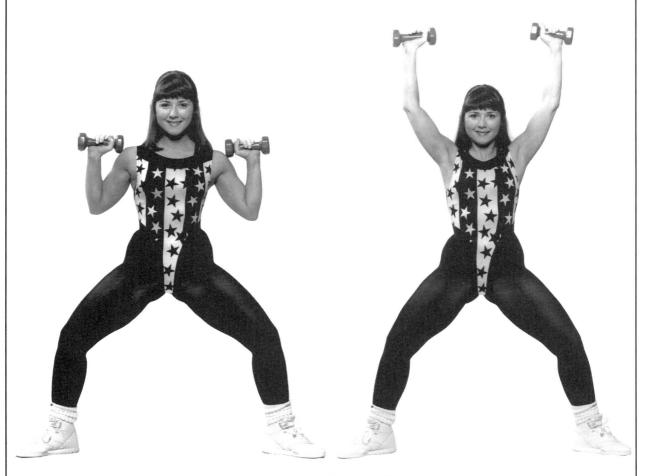

Position One: Stand with your feet shoulder-width apart, knees slightly bent. Hold the weights on your shoulders, palms facing forward. Make sure you do not squeeze the weight.

Position Two: As you exhale reach your hands up above your head. Keep your neck long and tall. Inhale and slowly return to the starting position.

YOUR UPPER BODY

2. Shoulders (deltoids)

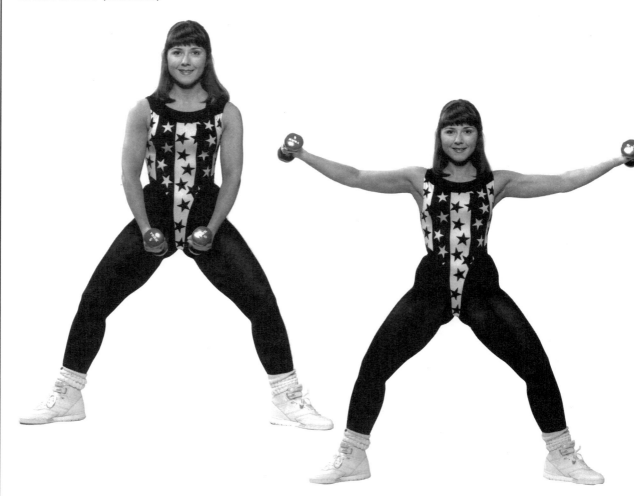

Position One: Stand with your feet shoulder-width apart, knees slightly bent. Hold the weights in front of your body, palms facing inwards, elbows soft.

Position Two: As you exhale, open your arms out to the sides. Stop when your hands reach shoulder level. As your arms raise, try to lengthen your neck and relax your shoulders.

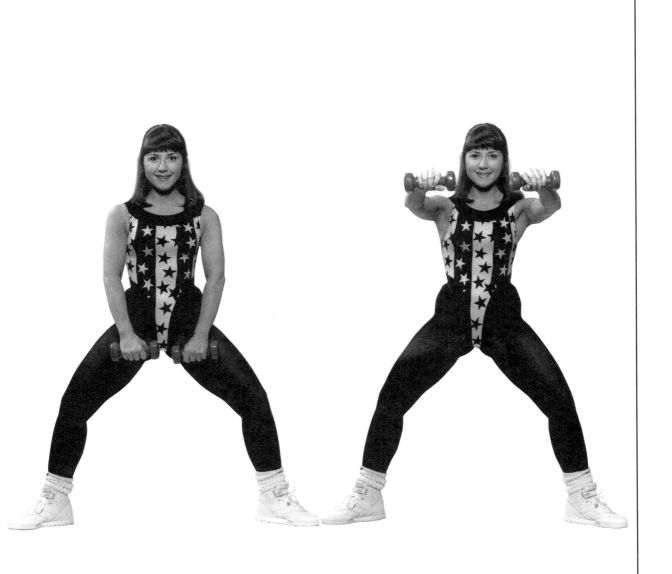

Position Three: Inhale and slowly lower your arms down in front of your thighs. Rotate your palms in so they face your body. Keep your ribs up high.

Position Four: As you exhale slowly lift your hands straight out in front of you, again stopping when you reach shoulder height. Inhale, slowly lower, and repeat the sequence.

YOUR UPPER BODY

3. Back of Waist (latissimus dorsi)

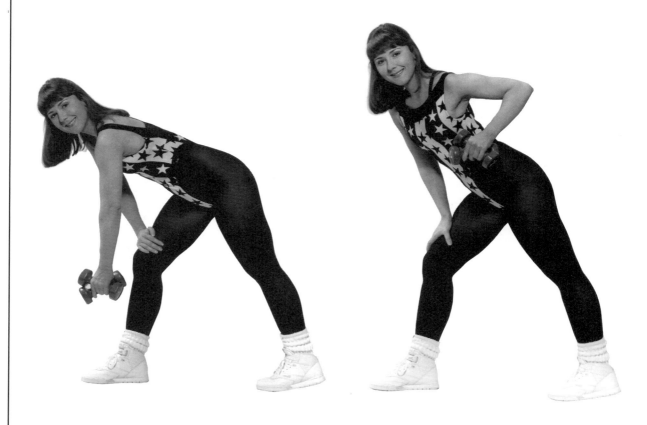

Position One: Stand with your right leg in front of the left, your right knee slightly bent. Lean on your right leg to support your back. Holding the weight in your left arm, allow the hand to hang down low to the floor. (Since this is a strong muscle group, you may double up your weights here.)

Position Two: As you exhale, bend your elbow and pull the weight up. Keep the elbow close into your waist as you lift. Imagine your shoulder blades coming together as your elbow points up. Inhale as you slowly lower and repeat. Then switch sides.

4. Front of Upper Arm (biceps)

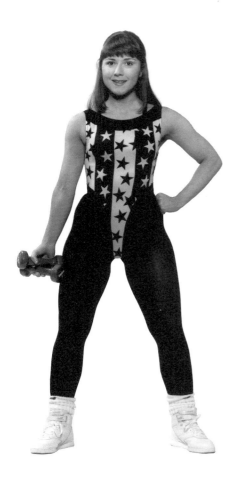 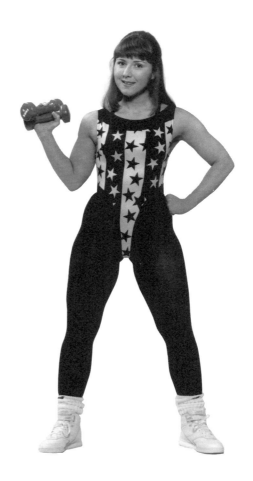

Position One: Stand or sit and hold your weights in your right hand. Keep your palm facing to the front and hold your arm on the side of your thigh. (Since this is a strong muscle group you may double up your weights here.)

Position Two: As you exhale, bend your elbow and lift the weights to your shoulder. Keep your palm facing forward throughout the entire lift. Inhale, lower and repeat. Then switch arms.

YOUR UPPER BODY

5. Shoulder Joint (rotator cuff muscles)

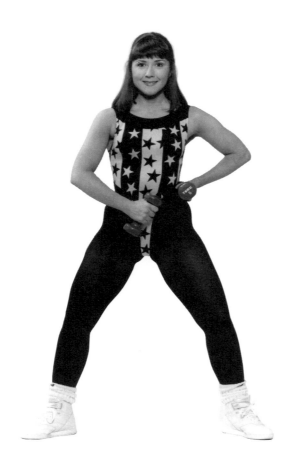 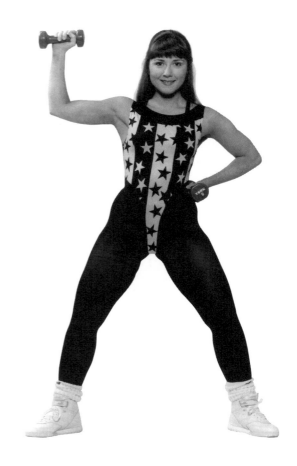

Position One: Using your lighter weights, hold your right hand in front of your abdomen, palm facing in. Keep your elbow slightly out to the side.

Position Two: As you exhale, slowly rotate your shoulder so that your hand raises up in front of you and stops when it is pointing to the ceiling. Hold, then lower very carefully. Repeat, then switch sides.

6. Back of Upper Arm (triceps)

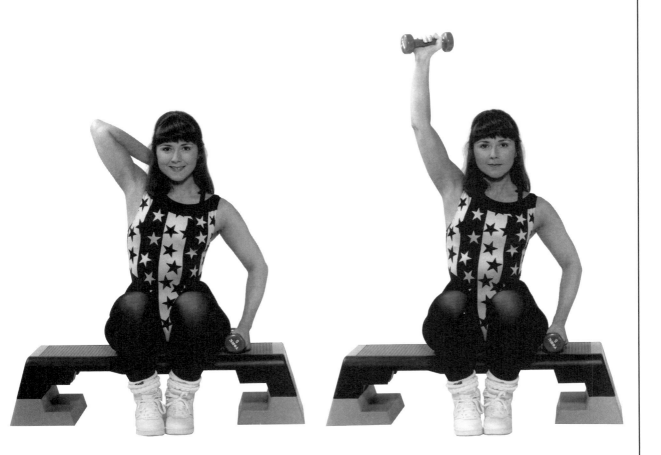

Position One: Sitting or standing, hold a weight in your right hand. Drop your hand behind your neck and point your elbow to the ceiling.

Position Two: As you exhale, keep your upper arm and elbow stationary while you lift your hand up to straighten your arm. Inhale, slowly lower and repeat.

YOUR UPPER BODY

7. Middle Back and Back of Shoulder (rhomboids and anterior deltoids)

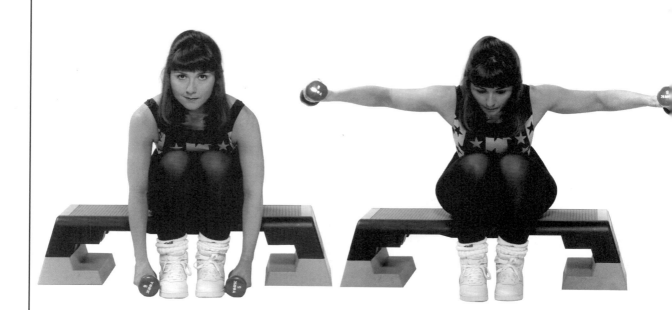

Position One: Sit on a bench or low stool, or if you only have a chair prop your feet up so that your knees are high enough to lean forward on. Rest your chest on your thighs and hold a weight in each hand by your feet, palms facing in.

Position Two: Drop your chin. Exhale and open your arms to the side. Remember to lean forward on to your legs so you work the back of your shoulders and back. If this feels uncomfortable use a light weight or bend your elbows a little when you lift.

8. Back and Shoulders (latissimus dorsi, rhomboids, deltoids)

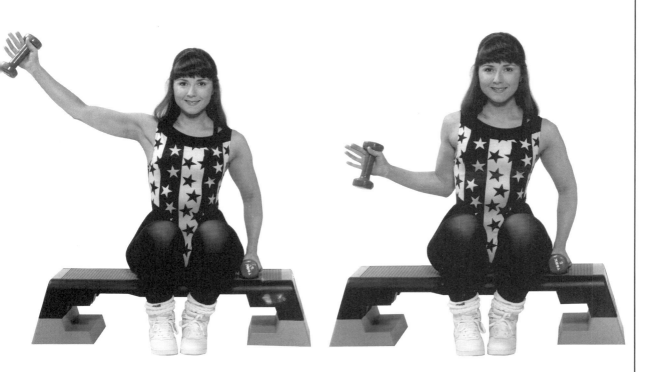

Position One: Sit or stand and hold a light weight in your right hand. Extend your arm so that your hand reaches up to the right corner where the wall and ceiling meet. Your palm is facing forwards.

Position Two: Pretend you are sliding the back of your right hand along a wall. Pull your elbow into your rib cage, keep your hand open to the side. Hold, repeat, then switch arms.

YOUR UPPER BODY

9. Chest (pectorals)

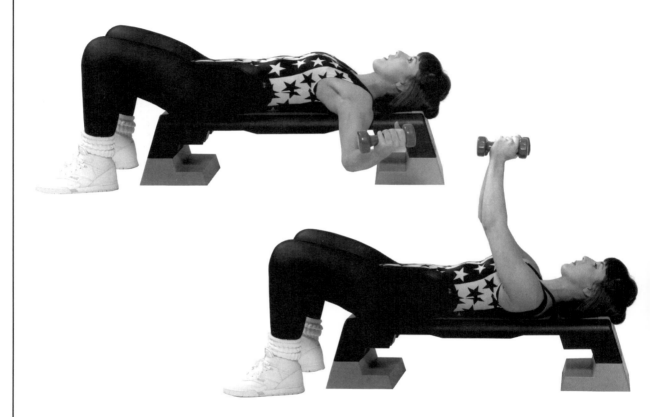

Position One: Lie on your back with your knees bent. Hold one weight in each hand and open your arms, dropping them slightly below your shoulders (if you are on a bench). Palms face up to the ceiling.

Position Two: As you exhale, squeeze your upper inner arms together so that your hands move out and up to meet about your chest. Inhale, slowly lower, then repeat.

YOUR LOWER BODY

10. Buttocks and Outer Thighs (gluteals, quadriceps and abductors)

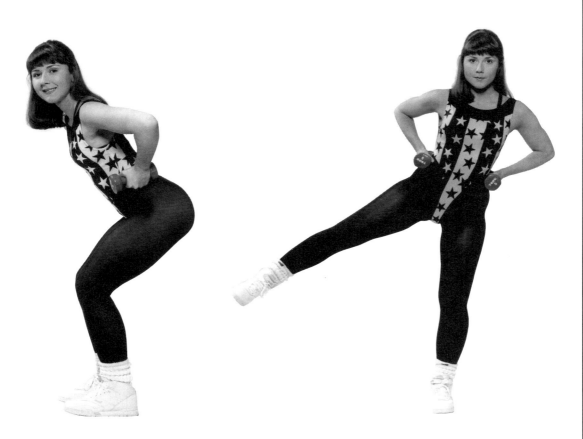

Position One: Stand with your feet parallel, shoulder-width apart. Keep your body weight in your heels, not toes. Tighten your abdominals and, with a straight back, lean at a slight angle forwards. Lower your hips as you push them out behind you. Do not tilt your pelvis forward but point your tailbone backwards. Hold the weights resting on your hips.

Position Two: With your body weight still in your heels, squeeze your buttocks and straighten your legs while you kick your right leg out to the side. Hold, then lower both legs into a squat again and repeat on the other leg. (Keep your straight knee facing front as you lift the leg).

YOUR LOWER BODY

11. Buttocks and Inner Thighs (gluteals, quadriceps and adductors)

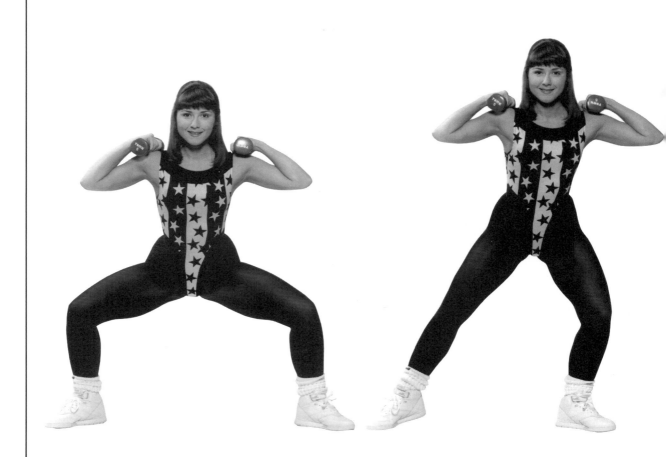

Position One: Hold your weights on your shoulders and stand in a wide straddle position with your knees bent. Your legs should form a square with your knees over your ankles. If your feet are too close, then your knees will jut forward over your toes. Open the feet wider if this is the case. Make sure your knees and toes point slightly out in the same direction.

Position Two: Press your right foot down into the floor and slowly drag it across towards your other leg. The foot pushing down provides extra resistance for your inner thighs as they work to close your thighs.

12. Back of Thighs and Buttocks (hamstrings, gluteals)

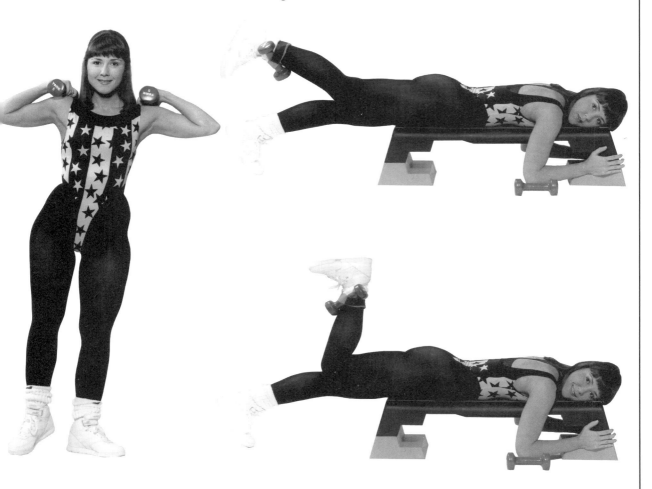

Position Three: Once your feet are together, open once again into a wide squat and press down into the floor and close with the other foot.

Position One: Lie on the floor or a bench on your stomach. If you have an ankle weight, strap it on. Extend your right leg and raise it two inches.

Position Two: As you exhale, bend your knee and bring your foot to your buttocks. Slowly straighten, lower your leg, then lift and repeat on the other side.

YOUR LOWER BODY

13. Lower Back (erector spinae)

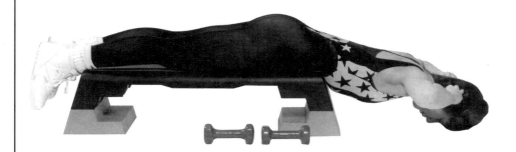

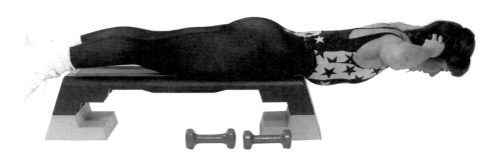

Position One: Lie on a step with your torso hanging over the top edge. Place your hands behind your head and keep your chin down.

Position Two: As you exhale, lift your back up to a horizontal position. Slowly lower, then repeat. (If you do not have a bench you may do this on the floor. Try to lift only one or two inches in this case.)

14. Back (erector spinae)

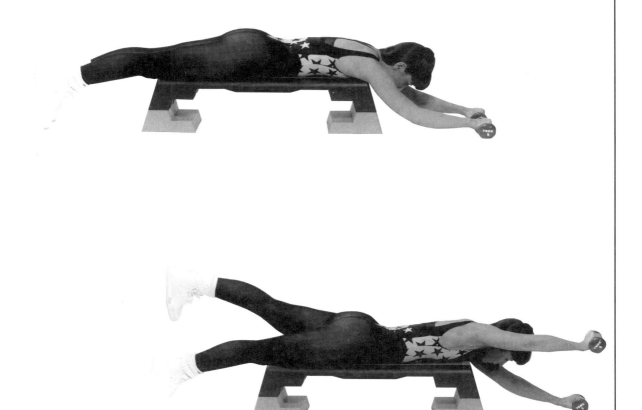

Position One: Lie on a bench or on the floor with your legs straight and your arms extended over your head. Hold a light weight in each hand.

Position Two: As you exhale, raise your right arm and left leg. Hold, lower, then repeat on the other side. Imagine you are drawing your shoulder blade down and across to the opposite hip.

YOUR LOWER BODY

15. Abdominals (rectus abdominus)

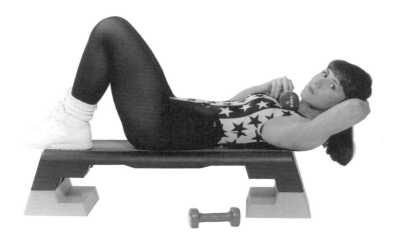

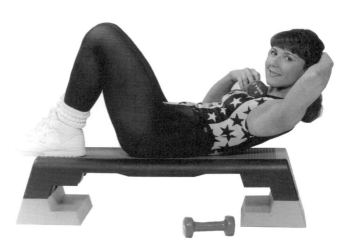

Position One: Lie on your back with one hand behind your head. Hold a weight just below your neck with the other hand. Keep your chin away from your chest.

Position Two: As you exhale, bring your ribcage towards your hips. Keep your chin open. Inhale and slowly lower so that your shoulder blades touch down but your head stays slightly lifted. Lift again. Change sides.

16. Abdominals (internal and external obliques)

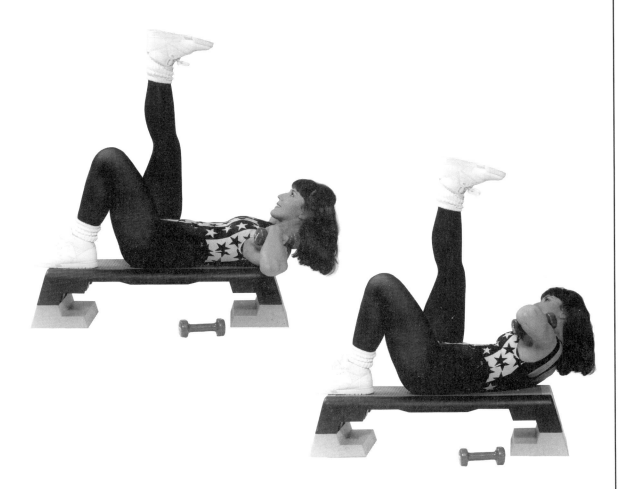

Position One: Hold a weight on your left shoulder and bring your right hand behind your head. Extend your right leg straight up, left knee bent.

Position Two: As you exhale, rotate your ribs so that your shoulder comes towards your opposite thigh. Hold, lower, then repeat. Change sides. Make sure you turn your ribs, not your neck.

YOUR LOWER BODY

17. Abdominals (rectus abdominus)

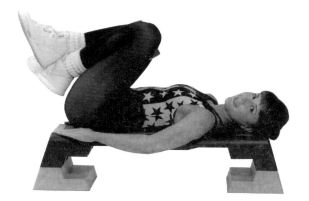

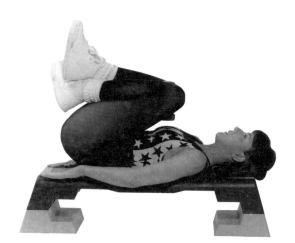

Position One: Lie on your back and bend your knees into your chest. Bring your hands by your hips for support.

Position Two: As you exhale, contract your abdominals and tilt your hips towards your lower ribs. Keep your knees into your chest. Hold, then slowly lower your tailbone. When you release avoid opening your thighs, keep them close into your body at all times. Try not to lift your back off the ground, just tilt your pelvis forward.

PART FOUR

STAYING MOTIVATED

CHAPTER 18

Continuing to Curve

So what happens next?

The next few chapters will show you how to stay motivated.

If you have completed your 12-week programme, you should be feeling much better than you did when you started. Depending upon which Curve you followed, you will have lost fat, increased your energy levels, improved your self confidence and/or become stronger. And, even better, you can continue to see or feel more improvements. The chances are, if you've stuck to it this long, the routine has become a habit and part of your lifestyle. It's easy for you to continue now because you expect to include activity in your daily routine rather than have to decide each day whether you will or not, giving yourself the opportunity to decide against. You've done well.

If you haven't completed your programme, then maybe you just need to give your motivation a jump start again. It's time to re-evaluate. Your needs are different now from when you started, so your programme should be too.

Keep Pushing On

Have you reached your goal? Certainly if your aim was to relax and feel more energetic, you probably did. But if you wanted to make significant changes to your body shape, the chances are you've made progress, but have not yet reached your goal. This is normal. Remember the changes take time: instantaneous body transformation just isn't possible. Congratulate yourself for completing your first 12 weeks. You have taken the most important step. Now you are ready to take the next one.

- *If you want to keep improving*, it is important to keep challenging your body. Remember, exercise is based on stressing various systems just enough so that they are forced to adapt to the demand. If you continued to perform at the exact same level and do the same amount of exercise, you would eventually cease to keep improving (although you would maintain your current level of fitness). To see further results you need to follow the Overload Curve and keep increasing the intensity in some way. This doesn't mean you have to work out harder and harder. You just need to manipulate your programme in different ways (re-read Chapter 6). You could add a new exercise to your regimen, or work out on an additional day each week. You could add an extra 10 minutes to your exercise session, or work out more intensely during the same amount of time. During the 12 weeks of your programme you will have already experienced the progressive overload of your workouts. Just continue in the same way.

Now that you have developed a good base level of fitness you can get slightly more specific with your programme. If you want to concentrate more on developing your upper body, consult a certified gym instructor for advice on a free-weights routine you can follow. Or if you want to try a new sport you are now fit enough to do so.

- *If you just want to maintain the point you have reached*, you can decrease your workload a little. As long as you continue at the same exercise *intensity* during your workouts, you can work out fewer times a week for shorter sessions. Studies have shown that only when the intensity at which you work is reduced will you have a measurable decline in your fitness level.

- *If the present level is still a challenge for you, or the pace is too fast*, continue at this level. Only increase the frequency, intensity or duration of your activities when they get too easy. Listen to your body and adjust your workouts accordingly.

Dropping Out

If you quit your programme mid-way through but are re-reading this to find out how to get back on track, go through the Body Transformation Strategy again and try to find out where you went wrong. Which activities were unsuitable or unmotivating?

What unexpected events prevented you from working out as much as you would have liked?

You know yourself a little better now. Evaluate how you felt when you started and how you felt when you stopped. Construct a regimen around the circumstances and personality traits you discovered the last time you attempted the plan. For example, if you scheduled evening fitness classes but never made them because you were too tired at the end of the day, try early morning workouts instead. If the idea of samba lessons appealed to you at first, but you then found them impossibly complicated, look for something just as much fun but less complex – nightclub dancing or cardiofunk, for example.

Stick To It

At the beginning of this book, I mentioned that there are a couple of mistakes that most people make. The first is not following the right fitness programme to reach your goal. The second is giving up too soon. Most people start off right, then, for whatever reason, stop before they realise the benefits

What Happens If I Stop Exercising?

The detraining effect depends on how fit you are to begin with and what type of exercise you usually do. The fitter you are to begin with, the fitter you'll be compared to less-fit counterparts if you stop training.

Cardiovascular fitness tends to develop quickly and deteriorate quickly. Muscular strength and endurance can last from two to four weeks of non-training after a period of building up your strength. But if you stop exercising after *short-term* training even just eight weeks of inactivity may put you back where you started.

Researchers at the University of Texas and the Washington University School of Medicine found that physical fitness in most people who stopped exercising declined rapidly in the first 12 days, and continued to decline thereafter, but not as quickly. However, even after three months of not exercising, these people were still measurably fitter than people who had never exercised.

Barbara had two children and was now in her mid-forties. Although she had been fairly active all her life, she had also always been overweight. She hired a personal trainer to visit her once a week. During those workouts she liked to work out at a high intensity doing aerobics, stepping and resistance exercises for an hour. She kept meaning to work out on other days but never managed to squeeze it in. Her husband (who was very fit) persuaded her to go to a health farm for three weeks. She lost some weight and exercised regularly. When she returned she fell back into her old routine. Her body shape returned to pre-health-farm levels. Finally, having worked with her trainer for a year, she gave up. Nothing seemed to work for her.

Lesson Her problem was that she simply did not exercise enough to achieve significant weight loss or changes in her body. It's easy to give up if you don't see results, that's why it's important to do as much as you safely can in the first few months of a body-shaping programme, then work on ways to overcome the excuses.

of their exercise. Being fit is like keeping your car in good condition: not only do you need to tune it up a few times during each year but you need to fill it up with gas, keep it clean and keep the systems functioning properly on a regular basis. If you don't it will wear and tear and eventually break down.

As we use more and more labour-saving devices, our activity levels are reduced accordingly. Exercise, therefore, is as necessary as brushing your teeth. It must be part of your lifestyle, not some temporary panacea or occasional whim. Whether you lasted this first 12 weeks or not, by now you will have realised that the hard part of the workout is not physical, but mental. The last two chapters are devoted to finding ways to keep you motivated to stick to your programme.

CHAPTER 19

Excuses

Your greatest ally and your greatest foe is your mind. Let's face it, you're capable of exercising. The difficult part is *continuing* to exercise and exercising when you just don't feel like it.

Exercise needs to become a habit, a normal part of your everyday life. It's dangerous to think of it in the short term because that implies it has an end in sight. If exercise is to create a lasting effect on your body it must be continued, to some extent, for ever. But that doesn't mean you are going to be living, breathing and dreaming exercise for the next fifty years. That would certainly be unrealistic but if you do a little bit consistently, then it is easy and it will help create the results you want.

Look upon your programme as a series of small tasks leading to a big project, otherwise you will be overwhelmed and intimidated and believe that the whole thing is hopeless and impossible. But the truth is, it isn't.

CONSISTENCY

It's easy to become obsessed for a short while and exercise every day for a couple of weeks. Many people seem to prefer giving an all-out effort for a short time. The problem is, whether you're dieting or exercising, your results won't be permanent unless you keep it up. From a practical viewpoint this obsession simply can't last without you having to neglect permanently other areas of your life. Eventually you'll spend time again on your work, relationships or social life. If you are

hoping to follow a compulsive few weeks of heavy exercise to achieve *and* maintain your goal, you are doomed to fail. On the other hand, if you gradually adopt more activity into your lifestyle you will actually exert less effort but show more and *more lasting* results.

It's all about consistency. Having a few days off or eating too much occasionally will not matter in the long term. It all balances out. If you were to eat an entire chocolate cake you wouldn't gain 10 pounds overnight, but if you ate a chocolate cake every day for a month you would gain weight. If you exercise very intensely for a few days and then stop, ultimately there will be little effect

---

Exercising in polluted air is worse than not exercising

Exercise makes you breathe faster and deeper, thereby increasing the air pollutants you inhale. The problem is worse in the summer on non-windy days, particularly in valleys. Bearing this in mind, work out in the early morning, choose areas with little traffic and breathe through your nose to help filter out some of the pollutants. Take notice of air ratings, and exercise inside on particularly bad days. If you have asthma or heart disease consult your doctor for advice on exercising.

on your body. If you exercise a little bit every day, ultimately there will be dramatic effects on your body.

THE TEN MOST COMMON EXCUSES AND HOW TO OVERCOME THEM

The whole point of the *Curves* strategy is to help you avoid becoming another drop-out statistic. Exercise works – if you stick to it. Dropping out is all too easy; it's tempting to postpone, give up or delay your workouts. In fact, most studies show that fifty per cent of all those who begin an exercise programme drop out within six months.

But if you want results your mind has to be as tough as your muscles to help you overcome the mental hurdles. Here are 10 tips to deal with the excuses so you won't become another statistic:

1. I'm Too Busy

Everyone uses this excuse, but studies have found that drop-outs had no less free time than their fitter counterparts! It's their priorities that are different. Keep exercise high on your list. Rather than telling yourself you'll work out when you get a chance, schedule it into each day. If you start out with good intentions but get sidetracked, exercise *early* so it's done and over with.

If you still can't squeeze it in, you can maintain your current fitness level by decreasing the frequency of your sessions providing you work at a higher intensity when you exercise.

2. Nothing Seems to Be Happening

Stop looking for a miracle, change takes time. The good news is that exercise can improve the way you look and feel. The bad news is that some people may have a harder time than others. Several studies have noted that stayers tended to have more fitness gains than drop-outs on an identical programme. The older you are, the slower the physiological adaptions take. But don't let that get you down: let it inspire you to be even more persistent.

For results, make sure you're doing the right thing. If you're trying to change your body shape significantly, you'll probably need to do endurance exercise like walking, running or aerobics at least five days a week. If you're just trying to improve your fitness level, you can stick to the standard three-times-a-week-for-30-minutes formula. If you are a beginner or work out at an easy fitness level, be aware that low-intensity workouts take longer to give results. Don't be disappointed, be patient.

3. I'm Exhausted

If you're tired, you're probably not going to feel much like doing *anything*. Sometimes exercise can wake you up. But if you're *really* tired, your body is susceptible to injury. Go to bed half an hour earlier or take naps to catch up on your sleep.

You may also feel tired and listless if you're not getting enough nutrients or calories to fuel your energy levels. Eat well so that your body functions efficiently.

4. I'm Depressed

Your mood can certainly determine how you feel about exercising. Many studies have shown that even a light exercise session can dramatically improve your mood. If you're angry or depressed, do *something*, even if it's just a short, brisk walk. Tell yourself that the exercise itself is what you look forward to, remind yourself you'll feel better afterwards.

5. I'm Unco-ordinated

The chances are you're not, you've just not learned the basic steps of an activity properly. Most types of exercise need some basic instruction as to safe technique. If you don't have a health club, sports centre or professional instructor nearby, find some books or videos presented by qualified experts.

If you took up an activity then realised your skill level needed to be reasonably developed before you could enjoy it, switch modes of exercise. Try something you can do *without* having to learn of lot of intricate movements first. Complex sports may be racket sports and golf. Easy sports are cycling and hiking. Martial arts, salsa dancing and ballet require lots of practice to get the moves right; aerobic dance or nightclub dancing are more flexible and allow you to work at a comfortable level.

6. I Can't Afford To Join A Health Club

Not everyone can afford a hi-tech health club. But not having access to a Stairmaster or indoor heated swimming pool isn't sufficient reason to give up. There are other ways to get an economical workout.

- Parks and streets are free. Walk or get together with friends to organise outdoor games.

- Exercise videos can provide you with a great workout for little money.

- Participate in charity fun runs, group walks or bicycle rides.

- Buy dumbbells, a step and a video. Invest in two sessions with a personal trainer to learn the technique, then follow the video. I've recommended some videos in Appendix B.

7. I'm Bored

Sometimes all you need is a change. Even wearing a new leotard can dramatically increase your motivation. Cross train – try different activities. Or if you need a big jump start go on a healthy holiday for a weekend. Try a health spa or hiking and biking trip.

8. I Slumped

Have you ever started a diet, gone off it in the morning and written off the rest of the day? It's natural to slip up and miss a few days in your schedule every now and then. It won't harm your long-term goal as long as your overall routine is consistent. If you are so rigid that you end up feeling guilty about taking time off, you'll end up obsessed and eventually give up. It's impossible to maintain perfection.

Turn your set-backs into something positive. Instead of berating yourself, give yourself feedback – figure out what caused the set-back and how you can prevent it happening again.

9. I Don't Like to Sweat

Your workout doesn't *have* to be strenuous. Harder workouts have a higher drop-out rate. Rather than going for regimented timetables, just aim to go from being less active to being more active. If you exercise very intensely for a few days and then stop, there will be little effect on your body. If you exercise a little bit every day, ultimately there will be dramatic effects.

10. I Have a Bad Back/Weak Knees

If you look for unrealistically quick results, you may do too much too soon, get injured and give up. If you develop an injury, try to find a similar substitute which doesn't aggravate it. Instead of running on a foot injury, swim. If your injury prevents you from exerting much effort, meditate or take a walk. Keep up an active lifestyle even if you have to lessen the activity itself.

CHAPTER 20

Work Out, Don't Drop Out

Forcing yourself to exercise is difficult. On the other hand, when you *want* to do it, it all becomes effortless. The key is keeping yourself motivated.

There is a certain phenomenon in aerobics classes which I call the `whoop factor'. Have you ever been in a class where the energy was vibrating, the music was fuelling the energy and for some reason it was all terrific fun and very exciting? Then suddenly, out of the blue, someone lets out a gigantic whoop, a noise which is unmistakably the sound of exuberant enjoyment?

Although you may not want to whoop uncontrollably while you're walking down the street, or mid-step while on the stairclimber machine, the idea is to make yourself *feel* like whooping. That way you'll know you enjoy your exercise enough to stick to it.

MOTIVATION STRATEGIES

1. Make the Conditions Conducive

Try to take into account every potential disruption in your routine. Decide today what time you will exercise tomorrow. Lay out your fitness gear so it's ready when you need it. Consider all the factors that may interfere (phone calls, appointments, eating times for instance) and be prepared to make a slight adjustment.

2. Different Days, Different Intensities

The amount of sleep you have had, your mood, diet and any stress you're under will affect your energy levels. Some days you'll feel stronger than others. Adapt your routine accordingly. Don't be afraid to take it easy, or even take a few days off. Avoid doing high-impact activities more often than three days a week.

3. Sleep

If you exercise when you're tired you will probably find that it wakes you up. But if you're *really* tired, take a nap instead. If you get adequate amounts of sleep, you will not actually have to motivate yourself. You'll have the natural energy and want to be active.

4. Eat Well

If you're not getting enough nutrients or calories, your body may not function efficiently and you'll feel tired and listless. Eat plenty of fruit, vegetables and other carbohydrates to fuel your energy levels.

5. Listen To Your Body

If you develop an injury, try to find a similar substitute which doesn't aggravate it. Instead of running on a sore foot, swim. If your injury prevents you exerting much effort, meditate or take a walk. It's very easy to focus outwards on your activity when you should be attuned to your physical sensations. Push yourself when you feel inspired, but rest when your body needs it. But avoid going overboard. Signs that you are working out too much include:

- Decreased appetite
- Difficulty sleeping
- Mood changes
- Increased injuries
- Impaired performance
- Constant fatigue
- Finishing exercise more tired than when you started

If this sounds like you, allow your body recovery time between workouts. Make sure you are getting enough sleep. Reduce the frequency of your workouts.

6. Variety

There are ways to keep variety in your workouts. You can switch to different activities. But you can also vary how you train during particular activities. If you walk regularly, some days you can walk slowly over a long distance, some days you may want to alternate walking with jogging, and other days you may want to focus on walking a mile as fast as possible. Sometimes you can utilise items in the environment to get you working harder: if you see steps, walk up and down them; walk backwards and sideways; walk up hills, and so on. Be creative!

7. Visualise

Many athletes strive for an altered state of consciousness where their senses are so attuned to the activity that it becomes effortless. Set aside five to ten minutes each day to visualise your exercise sessions. Breathe slowly and imagine yourself performing the activity. Try to reproduce the positive emotions and sensations associated with the activity and see yourself getting stronger, looking better. Concentrate on the image as much as possible. There is much research which suggests that visualisation can greatly enhance your performance. In fact many professional athletes swear by it.

8. Be Easy on Yourself

It's natural to slip up and miss a few days in your schedule every now and then. It won't harm your long-term goal as long as you are consistent overall. Be flexible.

9. Do Light Workouts Too

Numerous studies have shown that high-intensity exercise programmes have a higher drop-out rate. There are only 24 hours in a day: it's impossible to stick to a very time-consuming exercise regimen. You would simply end up neglecting other areas of your life. Try to incorporate more activity into your lifestyle but concentrate on being consistent, not excessive.

10. Be Realistic

Stop looking for a miracle. One study showed that those who stuck with their exercise programme saw it as a permanent change in lifestyle rather than a temporary solution and they expected to work out about three times a week. The drop-outs only expected to work out once a week. This alone would be enough to make most people quit since, the less exercise you do, the fewer benefits will be seen in a short time and this can discourage you from continuing.

If you are a beginner or work out at an easy fitness level, be aware that a low-intensity exercise takes longer to give results. Be patient. Results will come if you stick to it. If you're not satisfied with the results you're getting, re-evaluate your plan to see how you can make it more effective.

11. Seek an Aerobic High

Exercise releases pleasure hormones. To experience this is what is known as an `aerobic high'. This state can be attained only after about 60 minutes of intense exercise. If you've reached this point you could suddenly feel as if you're running on air and exerting no effort at all. If you are new to exercise you may not be capable yet of exercising at this intensity, but if you have built up a good base level of fitness, push yourself occasionally to reach this high.

12. Take Risks

Once you've established a routine, don't be afraid to veer off it occasionally to try new things. The fitter you become, the easier new activities will be for you.

13. Talk to Yourself Nicely

Instead of berating yourself for finishing your workout early, or even taking a day off, focus on what you've accomplished instead. Recognise the stages you'll go through. Initially you will have hopes of success, you will be enthusiastic and believe you can do it. As you become more experienced you'll start taking a more strategic perspective: in time you'll develop the confidence and toughness that will let you push yourself more.

14. Make a Public Commitment

Tell your friends and family what your goal is. Encourage them to encourage you if you're feeling unmotivated.

15. Chart Your Progress

I have had great success myself and with my personal clients when using a workout calendar. Each day you work out, fill in what you did: `ran 30' or `weights and step class'. Use a bright pink or yellow highlighter to colour in the square. Pretty soon you'll have a whole calendar filled with happy squares! If you find you have too many white squares you can immediately pinpoint your drop-out potential and start to rectify this. Some days, the fact that you're desperate to colour in a square is incentive enough to get you up off your bum and along to the gym.

16. Find a Partner

Plan to exercise with a friend. Even if at the last minute you don't feel like exercising, you're committed because he or she is waiting for you. Of course this isn't fool-proof. Once I met a friend in the park to go running. Neither of us was in the mood so we decided it was too cold and went for a pizza instead!

17. Do Your Best

You may not feel like doing your usual hour-long workout (or however long you plan to work out) on some days. Then don't. Cut the workout to 30 minutes but really push yourself during that time. Or just go for a long walk so at least you've done something. If you can just persuade yourself to do a little bit, you'll often find that you complete a whole workout anyway.

18. Entertain Yourself

Read a book or magazine or listen to a Walkman when you're on a stationary bike or stair machine. On your walk figure out what to do about a work or personal problem. Sometimes distraction is the best form of motivation, but make sure you are doing the exercise or activity correctly.

19. Convince Yourself

Running is a breeze, step classes are fun and easy: it's the getting yourself up off the sofa that is undeniably the hardest part. Engage yourself in a mental debate when you're feeling unmotivated and discuss all the reasons in favour of exercising. Remind yourself of your goal. Say it out loud. Then, before you can analyse yourself further, walk out the door and get started. Take one step at a time: every little one will help enhance your looks and improve the way you feel.

You now have the knowledge, the inspiration and the plan. Good luck with your body transformation!

Bibliography

Books

William McArdle, Frank Katch *and* Victor Katch, *Exercise Physiology: Energy, Nutrition and Human Performance*. Lea & Febiger, 1986.

American College of Sports Medicine, *Guidelines For Exercise Testing and Prescription*, 4th ed. Lea & Febiger, 1991.

Dorothy Harris PhD *and* Bette Harris EdD, *The Athlete's Guide to Sports Psychology: Mental Skills for Physical People*. Leisure Press, 1984.

Robert Nideffer, *Psyched to Win*. Leisure Press, 1992.

W. Jack Rejeski *and* Elizabeth A. Kenney, *Fitness Motivation: Preventing Participant Drop-out*. Human Kinetics, 1988.

Anthony Robbins, *Awaken the Giant Within*. Simon & Schuster, 1992.

Articles

'Medicine and science in sports and exercise', *Official Journal of the American College of Sports Medicine*, vol.26, no.5 (suppl.), May 1994.

The Berkeley Wellness Letter, University of California at Berkeley, June 1993.

The Berkeley Wellness Letter, University of California at Berkeley, January 1992.

Carlos Grilo PhD, Denise Wilfley PhD *and* Kelly Brownell, PhD, 'Physical activity and weight control: why is the link so strong?', *Weight Control Digest*, vol.2, no.3, May/June 1992.

Bryant Stamford PhD, 'Exercise can't always counteract your diet', *The Physician and Sportsmedicine*, vol.18, no.5, May 1990.

Steven N. Blair PEd, 'Weight loss through physical activity', *The Weight Control Digest*, vol.1, no.2, January/February 1991.

'Effects of exercise on female body-shape', *Australian Journal of Science and Medicine in Sport*, September 1991.

'Aerobic exercise and mood', *Sports Medicine*, vol.13, no.3, 160–170, 1992.

'Effect of habitual exercise on daily energy expenditure and metabolic rate during standardized activity', *American Journal of Clinical Nutrition*, vol.59, 13–9, 1994.

'Diet composition and postexercise energy balance', *American Journal of Clinical Nutrition*, vol.59, 975–9, 1994.

'Does the amount of endurance exercise in combination with weight training and a very low energy diet affect resting metabolic rate and body composition?', *American Journal of Clinical Nutrition*, vol.59, 1088–92, 1994.

'Exercise for the overweight patient', *The Physician and Sportsmedicine*, vol.18, no.7, July 1990.

Daniel Kosich, 'Aerobic and anaerobic', *IDEA Today*, Nov/Dec 1989.

Activities

Aerobic Machines

There are machines which will simulate just about every fitness activity. Most of them are computerised to help you adjust your fitness level and have graphics to keep you entertained. The most common machines in health clubs include: stair machines, rowers, stationary cycles (recumbent and upright), Versiclimber, Nordik trak/cross-country ski machine.

Aerobics and Fitness Classes

There are many different types of fitness classes so, before you decide you don't like aerobics, see what's on offer: aqua aerobics, cardiofunk aerobics, cardiosculpting aerobics, circuit training, conditioning, high-impact aerobics, low-impact aerobics, Pilates, slide aerobics and step aerobics are all listed alphabetically below.

Aqua Aerobics

Exercising to music in water is known as aqua aerobics. It is perfect for those who need the low-impact, supportive environment of the water. It is also quite fun but can be difficult to work at a very high intensity. Equipment such as resistance items and steps can also be used. Both conditioning exercises for the muscles and calorie-burning moves can be performed in the water.

Cardiofunk Aerobics

A form of low-impact aerobics with a funky dance rhythm. Although a good instructor makes it fun, it can be hard to follow. Those with back problems may find some of the moves too jarring.

Cardiosculpting Aerobics

A form of low-impact aerobics which incorporates standing leg exercises with low-impact movements. It is slow but intense, and not as 'dancy' as traditional aerobics. The intensive hip and thigh work add a conditioning element to this endurance workout.

Circuit Training

A type of fitness training that incorporates a variety of muscle conditioning exercises, such as squats, push-ups and upper-body moves, with aerobic activities such as step or jogging on the spot.

Conditioning

Traditional floor toning exercises condition underworked muscles. These exercises include leg lifts, squats, abdominal curls and push-ups. Ask an instructor for advice on proper technique and alignment. Conditioning exercises do not burn enough calories to reduce fat but will help make you firm. See also Resistance Training.

Cycling Outdoors

A low-impact activity. If you have knee problems, make sure the seat is high enough and the tension low. Riding outside on a bike where you have to bend forward may be stressful if you have back problems so try a more upright cycle if possible. Try to pedal with as many revolutions per minute as you can. Develops strong legs and is a good calorie-burning activity.

Dancing

Dancing includes anything from wild rap moves and disco to the more sedate ballroom dancing (although some of that can be quite strenuous too). Dancing develops endurance in your legs and improves your overall stamina.

Golf

Providing you don't use a cart, golf can give you a good workout since in the course of an 18-hole game you can burn a good number of calories. Good for stress too.

High-Impact Aerobics

Bad techniques and poor instruction are often responsible for injuries that occur while doing this form of exercise. High-impact aerobics should be done on a sprung wooden floor. You should wear a good pair of aerobic shoes. Foot patterns should be varied so that you do not land on the same part of the foot for a prolonged period of time. In other words, you are more likely to cause injury from repetitive stress if you jog on the spot for five minutes, do star jumps for five minutes and so on. Avoid jumps which go on for more than a few repetitions without alternating the repetitions. Limit aerobic activity to two to three times a week. A great way to eliminate some of the impact stress is to add low-impact exercises. Those with back, knee or ankle problems may wish to stick to a lower-impact activity.

Jogging – see Running/Jogging

Low-Impact Aerobics

This is less stressful because it eliminates much of the pounding done in high-impact aerobics. However, it too contains risks. Too many side-to-side movements strain the knees. Excessive arm movements cause pain to the shoulders and back. Avoid using hand weights during the class as they give little benefit and can cause shoulder or back injuries.

Martial Arts

There are a number of martial arts including Karate, Tai Kwon Do and Aikido. Some of the moves may stress your back, knees and other joints, but overall they provide an excellent workout.

Nordik Trak/Cross-Country Ski Machine

This machine works both your arms and legs. It can be difficult to learn to co-ordinate the movements but it is low impact and puts little strain on the body.

Pilates

Pilates is a method of stretching and conditioning which was originally developed by Joseph Pilates, a German, and based on his experience as a gymnast, boxer, martial arts instructor and body builder. The method uses apparatus to supplement the various floor exercises. Pilates movements are similar to basic stretch and conditioning exercises found in aerobics classes, yoga or even football training. The major difference is that, while general fitness classes focus on isolating each muscle so that it is worked and strengthened to its full capacity, Pilates rarely isolates one muscle group. Instead, two, three or four muscle groups are integrated in one motion. This is a sophisticated training technique. Initially, you need to be able to isolate each specific muscle but, once it has been strengthened, fluid movement requires that the the muscle groups chain together or co-ordinate each other.

Since the technique was originally geared for dancers, there is very definite emphasis on increasing strength in the inner thighs and abdominals. The development of somewhat exaggerated mobility in the joints – particularly the hips – and great flexibility in the muscles is encouraged: often the trainer pushes, flexes and extends your muscles for you. While this may be a requirement for a dancer or gymnast, the average person does not need that amount of flexibility and could be injured if it's not monitored well. So to be safe make sure that your Pilates teacher has a thorough understanding of muscle and joint biomechanics. The Pilates technique is not aerobic and therefore cannot strengthen the heart and lungs or burn enough calories to lose weight. But the importance of this slow, thoughtful movement is that it reduces stress. Pilates is a thinking exercise as it requires concentration and control.

Rebounding/Mini Trampolining

Exercising on a mini trampoline can give you a low-impact workout, although you need to make sure you move your arms and legs as vigorously as possible instead of merely bouncing. If the trampoline propels you into the air you can get a falsely elevated heart rate which would make it appear that you are working out harder than you actually are. This activity would be best for overweight people who are not used to high levels of activity. Walking may be more beneficial, however.

Recreational Sports

There are many activities, including rock climbing, kayaking/canoeing, rowing, sailing and skiing, which will give you a great workout. Because of the limited nature of their practice I have not included them in your programme. If you follow one of the Body Transformation Curves, however, you should develop a good base level of fitness to participate in these activities.

Resistance Training

Resistance training is just conditioning exercises with added resistance in the form of a weight or elastic band. This is the next step up from conditioning. Developing muscle mass improves your body shape. Those with arthritis or joint injuries often find that muscle strengthening relieves some of the stress from the weakened area. If you are just starting to lift weights, do so only under supervision. Weight training can improve your performance in other activities.

Rollerblading (also called inline skating)

Great for lower body muscular endurance and works the heart and lungs too. Stick to smooth surfaces and practise stopping. Can burn lots of calories.

Rowing

Usually done on indoor machines. Great for endurance and upper-body and leg conditioning. Can exacerbate back problems. Try to push off with your feet so that you feel resistance when you pull.

Running/Jogging

Run at a pace that feels right for you and walk whenever you feel the intensity is too much. Helps develop leg strength and aerobic fitness and burns lots of calories. You can run outdoors or indoors on a treadmill, but when running outside watch the surface. Though jogging has been given a bad press since the early craze, it is perfectly safe and one of the most natural forms of movement provided you wear good running shoes, are on a soft surface (ground rather than concrete) and limit your activity to no more than three or four times a week. Those with joint problems may wish to substitute brisk walking instead. Running on a treadmill allows you to adjust the speed and sometimes the incline so you can simulate running up and down hills.

Some believe that the pounding in running could damage a woman's internal organs. This is not true. Providing you are properly prepared, running is safe for both men and women. However, vigorous running is risky for members of either sex who have not trained properly, wear inadequate shoes, run on a poor surface, and/or do not stretch and warm up before and after exercise.

Slide Aerobics

Slide is the newest trend in fitness. The exercise consists of lateral sliding movements performed on a smooth piece of plastic. It is said to be comparable to inline skating (also known as rollerblading). The exercise can give you a good workout, but your technique must be perfect or you could overstress the knee joints. There is still much research to be done on this activity, so avoid overdoing it.

Sports

Good for developing co-ordination and other skills. Some of the sports can give you a good workout although the risk of injury can be high since there are always factors you can't control – sudden turns and twists, bumping into other people, etc. Rather than rely on the sport to get you fit, get fit first, then play your sport.

Squash

A very intense activity which puts a little competition and fun back into a workout. Those with knee, back or ankle problems would be advised to stick to a more controlled form of movement since sudden twisting or bending could exacerbate any injuries.

Stair Machines

One of the most popular pieces of equipment in the gym. Stair machines are low impact but very calorie intensive. You should maintain a proper upright posture during your workout and you should stop after 15-20 minutes. There are three different models: one is the standard machine, the second is a more bouncy version, and the third is actually a treadmill of revolving stairs rather than just steps which move up and down. This one is the most intensive, but it can be difficult to work out on for extended periods.

Stationary Cycles (recumbent and upright)

There are two types of indoor cycle: the upright version places you in the traditional bike posture, the recumbent has you seated in a chair-like seat with a back support and your legs extended in front of you to pedal. If you have back, neck, shoulder or other problems which could be strained on a traditional bike, this may be more comfortable for you as this position works the muscles in your buttocks and hamstrings more than the upright cycle, which focuses more on your calves and quadriceps.

Indoor cycling may be more difficult than outdoor because there is less airflow and you may feel hotter. Also the resistance is likely to stay fairly consistent – you pedal non-stop – whereas outside you may have periods of gliding downhill.

Step Aerobics

An up up, down down movement using a raised platform. The workout is intense and relatively easy to follow. Make sure you start off with a beginners' step class because the moves can be too complex if you haven't learned the basic foot patterns first.

Swimming

Safe for all fitness levels except those suffering some back or shoulder injuries when excessive resistance and hyper-extension of the joints may exacerbate the pain. Good for posture development and flexibility. The water has a meditative effect, so it's great for combating stress.

Toning Tables

Toning tables, also known as 'passive exercise machines', were developed in the 1930s as a therapeutic tool for rehabilitation. Different versions perform different functions, but the essential principle is that you lie down and the machine moves your leg or some other body part. A couple of the machines merely pummel your bottom to 'break away cellulite'. In recent years the tables have come under scrutiny because they have entered the marketplace en masse, claiming to help you lose inches by toning the muscles and smoothing out the 'ripple effect' of cellulite on the hips and thighs. Several studies have measured the total metabolic cost of an exercise session and found it to be equivalent to that of the subject lying down watching TV! So passive motion exercise does not appear to be beneficial for increased calorific expenditure or losing weight. Most of the exercises would be better done without the machines. But for older people who don't like competition, don't like to sweat, would feel uncomfortable in exercise classes and probably wouldn't do anything else, the machines may help a bit. Even such small amounts of activity can have long-term health benefits.

Versiclimber

Many gyms have this machine, which simulates mountain climbing. You hold on to handles and step on foot pedals, then move your arms and legs as if you were climbing up a rope. It's low impact and a great calorie burner.

Video Workouts

You can get a good workout by following an exercise video if it is presented by a highly qualified instructor. See Appendix B for my recommendations.

Walking

Walking is a good way to lose weight because it is low impact and therefore easy on your joints. As it's a weight-bearing activity, you can burn a good number of calories if you walk for extended periods. Because the intensity is low you have to walk briskly and for some time to obtain substantial benefits. There are many walking variations you can do: you can walk up and down hills, walk backwards, take long strides and short strides, and pump your arms vigorously to vary the intensity. Using hand weights is not advisable as they don't increase the intensity much and could lead to shoulder injuries.

Water Running/Water Walking

It is possible to get a good workout in the water because the water, while supporting your body, resists your movement. There are special foam belts you can wear so that you can run in the deep end and keep afloat. Marathon runners often use these to train to give their bodies a rest from the usual impact. They are available at running stores or from one of the distributors listed in Appendix B.

Yoga

Since yoga is very slow and controlled it is perceived as a very gentle form of exercise. But don't be fooled: most yoga classes contain moves that can put incredible strain on the back, knees and neck. If you have problems in any of these areas avoid movements such as the cobra, the plough, any excessive knee bends or bending forward from the spine (especially while standing). A very peaceful activity, yoga can definitely help with stress and flexibility, but physiologically cannot burn enough calories to lose any noticeable amount of fat or weight.

Contacts and References

Contacts

Fitness Industry Association (FIA), Suite 3, Argent House, 103 Frimley Road, Camberley, Surrey GU15 2PP (tel. 01286 676275)

Association of Personal Trainers (APT), Suite 2, 8 Bedford Court, London WC2D 9OU (tel. 0171 837 1102)

The National Register of Personal Trainers, Cecil House, 52 St Andrew's Street, Hertford SG14 1JA (tel. 01992 504336)

Chartered Society of Physiotherapists, 14 Bedford Row, London WC1 (tel. 0171 242 1941)

Fitness Professionals Association (UEL), Longbridge Road, Dagenham, Essex RM8 2AS (tel: 0181 849 3567)

The Exercise Association of England, Unit 4, Angel Gate, 326 City Road, London EC1V 2PT (tel. 0171 278 0811)

Aquaaerobics, 143 White Hart Lane, Barnes, London SW13 0JP (tel. 0181 878 9868)

IDEA: The Association for Fitness Professionals, Suite 204, 6190 Cornerstone Court East, San Diego, California 92121-3773 (tel. 001 619 535 8979)

Aerobics & Fitness Association of America (AFAA), Suite 310, 15250 Ventura Blvd, Sherman Oaks, California 91403 (tel. 001 818 905 0040)

Recommended Books

Anita Bean, *The Complete Guide to Sports Nutrition*, A & C Black, 1993

Glenn Town *and* Todd Kearny, *Swim, Bike, Run*, Human Kinetics, 1994

James Gavin, *The Exercise Habit*, Leisure Press, 1992

Dr Roy E. Vartabedian *and* Kathy Matthews, *Nutripoints*, Grafton, 1990

Naomi Wolf, *The Beauty Myth*, Chatto & Windus, 1991

Shelly Bovey, *Being Fat is Not a Sin*, Pandora, 1989

Marilyn French, *The War Against Women*, Hamish Hamilton, 1992

Recommended Videos

Any fitness videos by the following instructors are recommended. All should be available at your local video store.

Darryl Preston
Carolan Brown
Jane Waller/Fitness Professionals Association
Karen Voight
Keli Roberts
Kathy Smith

Jane Fonda
YMCA (Y-Plan)
Libby Roberts (Shape Challenge videos)
Mr Motivator

For information on Martica K. Heaner's books and videos contact: Mind & Muscle, PO Box 363, London WC2H 9BW (tel. 0171 240 9861)

Recommended Retailers of Fitness Products

It can be difficult to find good-quality exercise equipment such as free weights and elastic bands. The following are reputable mail order fitness equipment distributors who sell good-quality merchandise.

Energy Express, 36 Beech Lane, Kislingbury, Northants NN7 4AL (tel. 01604 832 843)

Aspire Fitness Products, CASE Sportscare, 4 Sandown Cottage, London Road, Teynham, Kent ME9 9JE (tel. 01795 522 599)

Forza Fitness Equipment, Fourth Floor, Europe House, The World Trade Centre, London E1 9AA (tel. 0171 488 9488)

Recommended Healthy Holidays

Rather than just lie on the beach doing nothing, take a healthy holiday. Below are some exceptional vacations:

IN GREAT BRITAIN:

Health Spas

Champneys, New Court, Wigginton, Tring, Hertfordshire HP23 6HY (tel. 01442 86 3351) Henlow Grange House Farm, Coach Road, Henlow, Bedfordshire SG16 6DB (tel. 01462 811111)

Hoar Cross Hall, Hoar Cross, Near Yoxall, Staffordshire DE13 8QS (tel. 01283 75671)

Thorneyholme Hall Health Spa, Dunsop Bridge, Clitheroe, Lancashire BB7 3BB (tel. 01200 8271)

Ragdale Hall, Ragdale, Near Melton Mowbray, Leicester LE14 2PB (tel. 01664 434411)

Chewton Glen Hotel, New Milton, Hampshire BH25 6QS (tel. 01425 275341)

Sopwell House Hotel and Country Club, Cottonmill Lane, Sopwell, St Albans, Hertfordshire AL1 2HQ (tel. 01727 864477)

Activity Breaks

Windmill Hill Place Tennis and Golf Resort, Windmill Hill, Near Hailsham, East Sussex BN27 4RZ (tel. 01323 832552)

Country Lanes Bicycle Tours, 9 Shaftesbury Street, Fordingbridge, Hampshire SP6 1JF (tel. 01425 655022)

The Centrecourt Hotel and Tennis Centre, Centre Drive, Chineham, Basingstoke, Hampshire RG24 0FY (tel. 01256 816664)

Gleneagles Hotel, Auchterarder, Perthshire PH3 1BR, Scotland (tel. 01764 62231)

ELSEWHERE:
Barringtons Heath and Leisure Club, Val Do Lobo, 8135 Almancil, Algarve, Portugal (tel 010351 893 96622)

The Phoenician, 600 East Camelback Road, Scottsdale, Arizona USA 85251 (tel. 0101 602 941 8200)

Canyon Ranch, Bellefontaine, Kemble Street, Lenox, Massachusetts 01240 *or* 8600 East Rockcliff Road, Tucson, Arizona USA 85715 (tel. 0101 602 742 9000)

Evian Health Spa, Royal Club Evian, Institute Mieux Vivre, Chteau de Blonay BP 877 4502.

Evian-les-Bains, Cedex, France (tel. 010 33 50 26 8500)

Butterfield and Robinson (biking and hiking around the world), 70 Bond Street, Toronto, Ontario, Canada M5B 1X3 (tel. 0101 416 864 1354)

Corijo Romero (Spain), Wendy Moffatt, 24 Grange Avenue, Chapeltown, Leeds, West Yorkshire LS7 4EJ (tel. 01132 374015)

Skyros Institute (Greece), 92 Prince of Wales Road, London NW5 3NE (tel. 0171 267 4424)
Backroads Bicycle Tours (around the world), 1516 5th Street, Suite Q333, Berkeley, California 94710-1740 (tel. 0101 510 527 1555) *or* 9 Shaftesbury Street, Fordingbridge, Hampshire SP6 1JF (tel. 01425 655 022)

Innactive Holidays (around the world), Inntravel, The Old Station, Helmsley, York YO6 5BZ (tel. 01439 71111)

Index